NEUROSCIENCE RESEARCH PROGRESS

NON-PHARMACOLOGICAL THERAPIES IN DIFFERENT TYPES OF DEMENTIA AND MILD COGNITIVE IMPAIRMENT

A WIDE PERSPECTIVE FROM THEORY TO PRACTICE

NEUROSCIENCE RESEARCH PROGRESS

Additional books in this series can be found on Nova's website
under the Series tab.

Additional e-books in this series can be found on Nova's website
under the e-book tab.

NEUROSCIENCE RESEARCH PROGRESS

NON-PHARMACOLOGICAL THERAPIES IN DIFFERENT TYPES OF DEMENTIA AND MILD COGNITIVE IMPAIRMENT

A WIDE PERSPECTIVE FROM THEORY TO PRACTICE

ELISABETTA FARINA
EDITOR

New York

Library of Congress Cataloging-in-Publication Data

ISBN: 978-1-63321-860-4

Library of Congress Control Number: 2014948651

Published by Nova Science Publishers, Inc. † New York

Contents

Preface **vii**

Chapter 1 Evaluating Oral Reading and Reading Comprehension in Patients with Dementia: A Comparison of Generic and Personally Relevant Stimuli **1**
Jeanette E. Benigas and Michelle S. Bourgeois

Chapter 2 Exploring the Use of Two Different Gardens by Residents in a Special Care Unit for People with Dementia **15**
Antonio Guaita, Erminia Gadler, Giovanni Andreoni, Marinella Mancuso, Riccardo Perelli Cippo, Chiara Cutaia, Mauro Colombo and Silvia Vitali

Chapter 3 Practical Protocol for Implementing Cognitive Stimulation in Persons with Delirium Superimposed on Dementia **31**
Ann M. Kolanowski, Nikki Hill, Linda Clare and Patricia Marx

Chapter 4 How Do People with Dementia and Their Carers Evaluate the Meeting Centers Support Programme? **41**
Rose-Marie Dröes, Franka J. M. Meiland, Mirjam J. Schmitz and Willem van Tilburg

Chapter 5 Pilot Study Protocol of an Educational Intervention for Caregivers of People with Psychological and Behavioral Symptoms Due to Dementia **63**
S. F. Vitali, C. Cutaia and R. Vaccaro

Chapter 6 The Additional Contribution of Combination of Pharmacological Therapy and Cognitive Stimulation in Alzheimer's Disease: Review of the Literature **73**
Maria Cotelli, Rosa Manenti and Orazio Zanetti

Chapter 7	Cognitive Rehabilitation in Mild Cognitive Impairment: A Pilot Study *Elena Farini, Paola Frasson, Giada Caramatti, Eleonora Catricalà, Jubin Abutalebi, Alessandra Marcone and Stefano F. Cappa*	**83**
Chapter 8	From Smartphone to External Semantic Memory Device: The Use of New Technologies to Compensate for Semantic Deficits *Sonia Routhier, Joël Macoir, Hélène Imbeault, Séverine Jacques, Hélène Pigot, Sylvain Giroux, Albert Cau and Nathalie Bier*	**93**
Chapter 9	Effectiveness (or Not?) of Cognitive Rehabilitation in a Person with Semantic Dementia *Fabiana Villanelli, Annamaria Russo, Raffaello Nemni and Elisabetta Farina*	**113**
Chapter 10	Impact of Non Pharmacologic Interventions on People with Dementia and Their Caregivers: A French Perspective *Florence Bonté*	**121**
Index		**129**

Preface

This book presents current research in the study of non-pharmacological treatment proposed in dementia care. Topics discussed include cognitive stimulation and rehabilitation, oral and reading comprehension, new technologies, educational intervention for caregivers, and contributions of pharmacological therapies.

Chapter 1 – The purpose of this study was to compare the reading comprehension performance of persons with dementia (N = 20) using personal and generic stimuli. Each subject participated in two data collection sessions over a 7-day period. Subjects were presented with five generic and five personal stimulus pages and were prompted to "Read this sentence and tell me something about it." Results indicated that subjects' reading accuracy was consistent over a 7-day period, and that, more novel comments overall and more novel comments indicating reading comprehension were made with personal stimuli when compared to generic stimuli. Personal stimuli may have advantages over generic stimuli for enhancing reading comprehension and communication in persons with dementia.

Chapter 2 – *Backgrounds.* The purpose of this study is to examine the use of two different Alzheimer's gardens, one designed as a "quiet space" and the other as an "activity" garden, by direct observations of behavior of the forty two residents in a Special Care Unit for people with dementia.

Methods. Observations were conducted within the gardens to evaluate whether they were used by residents and how, including frequency of visit, way in which the gardens were used for individual and social activities. Since residents are persons with dementia with clinically diagnosed Alzheimer disease, other dementias or psychosis, the authors compared the recorded behaviors of these three groups.

Results. Findings suggest that the two gardens are used differently in the activities performed according to gender, diagnosis and garden characteristics, while frequency is different only for the time of the day.

Conclusion. These data confirm the importance of the connection between persons with dementia and environment, that can be considered essential part of the therapeutic protocol.

Chapter 3 – Delirium is common in persons with dementia and often accompanies acute medical or surgical conditions. These individuals are at risk for an accelerated decline in their cognitive and physical function. For this reason, interventions that help resolve delirium are critically needed. The authors have developed a non-pharmacological intervention for delirium in persons with dementia based on their prior interdisciplinary work on delirium, dementia and cognitive stimulation. The intervention uses recreational activities that are alerting, capture attention, and provide cognitive stimulation that encourages cognitive processing in support of cognitive function. In this paper the authors describe the practical protocol they have developed for implementing these activities, and present a video that will enhance treatment fidelity for studies that replicate the approach.

Chapter 4 – *Background.* The Meeting Centers Support Programme (MCSP) offers information and practical, emotional and social support to persons with dementia and their carers in local community centers. In this study the support programme was evaluated by participants (persons with dementia and carers) who utilized the MCSP for at least three months.

Methods. Data collection took place within the framework of an implementation study in 11 meeting centers. 148 persons with dementia and 148 carers participated in the study. Data were collected after three and seven months of participation by means of questionnaires.

Results. In general the persons with dementia and the carers were satisfied to very satisfied with the different elements of the support programme, the enrolment procedure, the contact with personnel, the location, and the facilities the centers have to offer. Half of the persons with dementia and one third of all carers indicated that they had made new acquaintances and friends at the center. Though satisfied with the programme, a majority of the persons with dementia (67% after three months and 58% after seven months) said that they were never asked what they wanted to do. The large majority of the carers feel somewhat less (42%) or much less (46%) burdened as a result of participating in the programme. This reduction of experienced burden proved to be related to satisfaction about the total programme (r_s=0.35, $p<0.005$), experienced understanding for the own situation in informative meetings (r_s=0.19, p= 0.05), and experienced emotional support in contacts with other carers (r_s=0.19, p=0.03).

Conclusion. The satisfaction of the persons with dementia and their carers about the MCSP, and the percentage of carers who experienced a reduction of burden thanks to the support they received are high. However, the fact that two thirds of the persons with dementia say that they were never asked what they want to do indicates that the methods used by the staff need to be improved.

Chapter 5 – The purpose of the study is to describe an educational program for caregivers of people with dementia and behavioral-psychological symptoms (BPSD), admitted to the Special Care Unit (SCU) of the authors' Institute for a temporary stay. The prosthetic approach used in the SCU considers informal caregivers (families) as partner of the formal ones (staff) in building up the program of care.

The intervention is aimed at extending to the caregivers an interpretative approach to the BPSD, and at sharing with them the results of a systematic approach used from the staff to understand the possible causes of these symptoms.

The core of the intervention is based first on training the family in learning ABC (antecedents-behavior-consequences) approach to assess and monitor the PWD (person with dementia) behaviors, then on training and supporting caregivers to apply the suggested interventions.

At the same time caregiving issues appearing during the period of their stay in the unit are addressed in a therapeutically alliance with the family. The hypothesis author's assume is that this practice will be able to enhance caregivers ability to manage critical situation in the care process. Outcome measures will be caregivers self efficacy and stress measures.

Chapter 6 – Alzheimer's disease (AD) is a progressive disorder that impacts several cognitive functions. However, some aspects of cognitive function are preserved until later in the disease and can therefore be the targets of specific interventions. The rehabilitation of cognitive function disorders represents an expanding area of neurological rehabilitation and it has recently attracted growing political, social and ethical attention. Here author review the efficacy of combining cognitive stimulation and cholinesterase inhibitors. Generally, all the studies reported in this review have compared the combined treatment with pharmacological intervention alone. Further studies should clarify the potential role of the combined cognitive-pharmacological treatment in AD persons with dementias care. In the meantime, the findings of the studies reviewed in this paper suggest that cognitive rehabilitation should be an essential part of dementia treatment, along with anti-dementia drugs.

Chapter 7 – *Introduction.* There is some evidence that cognitive rehabilitation can delay cognitive and functional decline in healthy older adults and person living with Alzheimer's disease (AD). Persons living with mild cognitive impairment (MCI) usually retain a wide range of cognitive capacities, and may thus represent an ideal target for cognitive rehabilitation.

Aim. To investigate the effectiveness of a 8-week cognitive rehabilitation program in persons living with MCI.

Subjects and methods. The study included an experimental group of 10 subjects (5 with Amnestic MCI -a-MCI- and 5 with amnestic multi-domain MCI -amd-MCI) and a control group of 5 comparable subjects (2 with a-MCI and 3 with amd-MCI). The experimental and control group were matched for Mini Mental State Examination (MMSE) score, years of education, age, basic activities of daily living (BADL), and instrumental activities of daily living (IADL). The rehabilitation program included a computerized cognitive rehabilitation program, drills with graded levels of difficulty, homework and specific instructions about the use of the strategies in real-life situations.

Results. The study outcome measures were the scores on neuropsychological tests as well as the functional status (IADL, BADL), which were assessed prior to enrolment, at the end of the rehabilitation program and after 2 months. In the experimental group the 2 months follow-up assessment revealed no significant differences in neuropsychological tests, except for a significant improvement in phonemic verbal fluency. In contrast, the controls showed a worsening of performance in semantic and phonemic verbal fluency and in IADL at the time of the third evaluation, two months after the end of treatment. One of the trained MCI and 3 out of 5 control subjects progressed to AD during the period of the study.

Conclusion. The results of this pilot study suggest that a comprehensive cognitive rehabilitation program may have beneficial effects on cognitive function and functional status in both a-MCI and amd-MCI subjects.

Chapter 8 – *Background:* Semantic dementia (SD) is a neurodegenerative disorder characterized by a progressive loss of semantic memory. The components of SD include impaired word comprehension, anomia and difficulties retrieving people's names. To date, most interventions aimed at improving language-based performances (e.g., naming) and often led to modest results. However, people living with SD could benefit from an ecological intervention focusing on compensation for their needs in activities of daily living (ADL). The use of new technologies is an interesting way to achieve such a compensatory approach for ADL in SD.

Aims: The aim of this case study was to investigate the effectiveness of an ecological compensatory and technological intervention in SD rehabilitation. More specifically, the goals were to help a person suffering from SD via the use of a smartphone (1) to retrieve people's names, and (2) to find semantic information essential to comprehension and naming.

Methods: ND is a 51 year-old man who has suffered from SD for 5 years. At baseline, daily self-report measures were used to document the number of times he could not retrieve a person's name and the number of times he used a paper notebook with personal clues to retrieve a name. The number of times he used a paper dictionary to find semantic information essential to comprehension and naming was also measured. The paper notebook and paper dictionary were two self-developed compensatory strategies. The intervention consisted of introducing a smartphone equipped with a new application called ARCUS and with Internet access. ARCUS is a virtual name directory allowing searching for names using personal cues. Daily self-report measures were taken for 2 months after the introduction of the device to measure concurrent use of the smartphone and the previous self-developed compensatory strategies.

Results: A sharp increase in the general tendency to compensate for name-finding difficulties was noted after the introduction of the smartphone. A large general preference for the smartphone over the paper notebook and paper dictionary was also found. The effectiveness of the smartphone and its ease of use were also very satisfactory.

Conclusion: New technologies such as smartphones can be an efficient compensatory intervention in SD. Focusing on the person's needs, the smartphone allowed ND to efficiently compensate for his difficulties in retrieving people's names and to find semantic information essential to word comprehension and naming. New technologies may have a central role to play in SD rehabilitation by providing a fast, efficient, mobile, accessible, ecological and non-stigmatizing way to compensate for deficits.

Chapter 9 – The authors tested the possible efficacy of relearning ecologically relevant information and its maintenance in Marian, a person affected by Semantic Dementia (SD).

In Phase 1, 20 images, belonging to two different categories of objects (vegetables and fruit), have been chosen among the ones Marian did not recognize: in each category, 5 have been used for the 2 month training (twice a week) with explicit and implicit memory techniques while the other 5 haven't. Statistical analysis comparing *trained-not trained* words at the end of the rehabilitation period was not significant, even if a slightly better performance in rehabilitated words was evident. At 6 months follow-up no training gain was evident.

In Phase 2, the authors performed a repeated baseline assessment and then they introduced a photo-vocabulary, which included 14 relatives' names. At baseline, Marian constantly denominated 1 relative only. In this second phase, Marian both followed structured rehabilitation sessions and rehearsed face-name associations at home. After two months Marian named 8/14 relatives (14/14 after phonemic cue). At 6 months follow-up, she spontaneously named 11/14 relatives' names (14/14 after phonemic cue).

In the second training phase, Marian showed a clearer improvement. This better result could depend on the fact that relatives' identification was less affected than identification of different kinds of food, or on the intensiveness of training or on Marian's better motivation.

The progression of the disease, however, stopped the authors from further treating Marian. Therefore, as shown by other Authors, a cognitive rehabilitation training based on relearning with explicit and implicit memory techniques seems to show a limited effectiveness in SD.

Chapter 10 – The article briefly describes the characteristics of the geriatric care organization in France, and in particular the role of medium term Day care Hospital (DCH) and the personal experience of the Author in this setting. People with dementia admitted in medium term DCH are sent by specialists from the memory clinic, short term DCH, or general practitioners (GP), simply because of the need of rehabilitation or in case of a sudden crisis at home. In this setting, non-pharmacological therapies, among these Art and Music therapy, can be delivered to people with dementia, while their caregivers can receive information and support.

In: Non-Pharmacological Therapies ...
Editor: Elisabetta Farina
ISBN: 978-1-63321-860-4

Chapter 1

Evaluating Oral Reading and Reading Comprehension in Patients with Dementia: A Comparison of Generic and Personally Relevant Stimuli

Jeanette E. Benigas and Michelle S. Bourgeois*
University of South Florida, Department of Communication Sciences and Disorders
Tampa, Florida, US

Abstract

The purpose of this study was to compare the reading comprehension performance of persons with dementia (N = 20) using personal and generic stimuli. Each subject participated in two data collection sessions over a 7-day period. Subjects were presented with five generic and five personal stimulus pages and were prompted to "Read this sentence and tell me something about it." Results indicated that subjects' reading accuracy was consistent over a 7-day period, and that, more novel comments overall and more novel comments indicating reading comprehension were made with personal stimuli when compared to generic stimuli. Personal stimuli may have advantages over generic stimuli for enhancing reading comprehension and communication in persons with dementia.

Keywords: Persons with dementia, reading comprehension in dementia, communication in dementia

Introduction

Nursing home residents with dementia have cognitive impairments that make communication with caregivers difficult. Memory problems, such as difficulty encoding, registering and learning new information, storing information (e.g., remembering what was

* Corresponding author: Michelle S. Bourgeois, Ph.D., CCC-SLP, Professor, University of South Florida, Department of Communication Sciences and Disorders, 4202 E. Fowler Ave., PCD 1017 Tampa, Florida, 33620. Phone: 813.974.9778 & E-mail: msbourgeois@usf.edu

eaten at breakfast), and information retrieval (e.g., remembering words and names) are common (Baddeley, 1995). As neurologic disease progresses, mild word-finding problems during conversation make utterances inaccurate, repetitious, and "empty." In the end stages, mutism and social withdrawal prevent satisfactory social interactions (Bourgeois and Hickey, 2009). These memory-related communication deficits often result in depression on the part of the person with dementia and their caregivers, reluctance to interact with caregivers, the inability to get wants and needs met and to communicate preferences, and a decrease in socialization.

Memory aids, such as memory books and memory wallets have been developed to help improve communicative interactions with nursing home staff and loved ones, in addition to improving the overall quality of life in people with dementia (Bourgeois, 1992a, 1993; Bourgeois and Mason, 1996; Hoerster, Hickey and Bourgeois, 2001). Memory books provide pictures and sentences for people to use to access facts and episodic memories for conversation. Bourgeois and colleagues have found that memory aids were successful for improving conversational interactions with familiar communication partners across a variety of settings (Bourgeois, 2007).When the individuals used the memory aid by reading the written sentences and describing the illustrations, the number of on-topic utterances and statements of fact increased, the number of off-topic utterances decreased, and conversational turn taking improved. These findings were replicated with persons with dementia of varying severities when the memory aid was modified to ensure the person could see the pictures and read the sentences (Bourgeois, 1992a). Enlarging the font size of the text and the size of the pictures allowed persons with declining vision and attention to be able to use the memory aid to access information from memory for conversations.

In order to determine the appropriate size of visual stimuli for an effective memory aid, clinicians need to evaluate the reading skills of the person with dementia. Dementia-specific reading measures, however, are limited. The *Bourgeois Oral Reading Screen* (BORS; Bourgeois, 1992b) was developed to assess oral reading performance with two font sizes in order to select the most appropriate font size for the person's memory book. This measure consists of five items, with one sentence and illustration on each page. The sentences are four - six word, simple, declarative sentences, written in the first person (e.g., "I enjoy baseball games;" "My sister is 75 years old."). The pictures are clipart line drawings. The five items are printed in either 18 pt. or 42 pt. Times New Roman font, and are presented to the person to read in a 3x5 inch or an 8x11 inch notebook. To score the measure, each correctly read word is counted (a total of 24 words); 90% oral reading accuracy determines optimum font size.

While the *BORS* was useful for determining appropriate font size for oral reading, clinicians questioned the degree to which persons with dementia comprehended what they read aloud. Standardized reading comprehension measures for people with dementia are limited to single word and sentence comprehension using picture choice tasks (Bayles and Tomoeda, 1993, 1994). People with dementia often demonstrate impaired reading ability on these subtests, in contrast to measured reading abilities on functional informal tasks. On standardized tests the complexity of the reading task, including the format of the expected response, might interfere with the demonstration of accurate reading comprehension. For example, the directions are presented verbally in a multi-step format; multiple stimuli (an array of picture or sentence choices) are involved; and a forced choice from the array is required. These features of the tasks require multiple cognitive processes, including memory for the instructions, visual discrimination of the features of the different response choices, and adequate executive functioning for decision-making.

Bourgeois and colleagues (2002) investigated the potential use of the *BORS* as a measure of reading comprehension after observing that people were making novel comments about the items after reading the sentence. For example, after reading the sentence, "My sister is 75 years old," the person might say, "I don't have a sister, only a couple of brothers." Transcripts from previous research (Bourgeois et al., 1999, 2000) were evaluated and it was discovered that subjects made comments suggesting comprehension for 20% of the stimulus items read aloud. Bourgeois and colleagues (2002) then conducted a pilot study to determine whether a prompt to comment about the read statement would increase the number of comments indicative of comprehension. Nine nursing home residents with dementia were asked to read the five sentences in the *BORS* and to make a comment about the statement. For 85% of the sentences read aloud, subjects made a comment that was judged to demonstrate comprehension of the statement.

In a follow-up study, Bourgeois and colleagues (2002) replicated these findings with another sample of 36 subjects with dementia who were also administered the word and sentence reading comprehension subtests of the *Reading Comprehension Battery for Aphasia (2nd* ed.) (RCBA-2; LaPointe and Horner, 1998) and the *Functional Linguistic Communication Inventory* (FLCI; Bayles and Tomoeda, 1994). Strong correlations were shown between comprehension on the *BORS* and the *RCBA* (.92) and between comprehension on the *BORS* and the *FLCI* (.90). These findings suggest that reading comprehension can be assessed during an oral reading task.

For many years researchers have observed that people with Alzheimer's-type dementia (AD) may have a preserved ability to read aloud word level material comprised of high frequency and regularly spelled words (Bayles et al., 1992) even into the late stages of the disease. In contrast, Patterson, Graham and Hodges (1994) have argued that this same population does not have a spared ability to read orally based on their evidence evaluating low-frequency words with irregular spelling-sound correspondences. The difference between high and low-frequency word reading may be related to how those words are stored in long-term memory and how they are accessed to perform a reading task.

Evidence of greater reading accuracy with regular and high frequency words was reported by Dietz and colleagues (2009). Individuals with chronic aphasia were asked to read narratives with either high-context photographs, low-context photographs or no-context (only the narrative) and then were asked a series of comprehension questions. Subjects who received the high-context photographs answered the highest number of questions correctly (Dietz et. al, 2009). These findings suggest that high-context visual stimuli, which are familiar and have been viewed more frequently when compared to low-context pictures, improve access to semantic memory where both words and pictures are stored resulting in evidence of reading comprehension. Similarly, the fact that memory books consisting of sentences and pictures about familiar topics contribute to improved access to semantic memories during conversation provides evidence of reading comprehension. Most standardized measures of reading comprehension and informal measures all use generic, non-familiar, sentences and pictures. It would be important to know if using familiar, high frequency stimuli would improve the reading comprehension performance of persons with dementia. Therefore, this study examined the reading comprehension performance of persons with dementia using stimuli consisting of familiar words and pictures. It was hypothesized that people with dementia would demonstrate greater comprehension of stimuli consisting of personally relevant information than generic information.

Methods

Subjects

Nursing home staff identified potential subjects for this study and provided the contact information for their power of attorney. Informed consent was obtained from the potential subject's power of attorney who also provided relevant photographs for the personal stimuli. The medical chart was reviewed to confirm the inclusion criteria including the diagnosis of dementia (e.g. dementia not otherwise specified, vascular dementia, Alzheimer's) and the absence of a focal lesion, transient ischemic attack or other psychiatric illness. Biographical and medical information were collected from the subject's medical chart.

Screening and data collection sessions were conducted sitting at a table in the subjects' rooms or in another quiet location within the skilled nursing facility. Outside noise was minimized to reduce distractions by turning off radios and televisions, pulling privacy curtains and closing doors. All sessions were audio recorded with an Olympus DS-40 digital voice recorder with timer. Subjects participated in one screening session of no more than 30-minutes in length and two data collection sessions within seven days which were 20-minutes or less in length.

The subjects were screened using the language, memory, and symbol cancellation subtests of the *Cognitive Linguistic Quick Test* (CLQT; Helm-Estabrooks, 2001), followed by the reading subtest of the *Wide Range Achievement Test,* 3rd ed. (WRAT-3; Stone, Jastak, and Wilkinson, 1995). Twenty-two patients were screened and 20 were enrolled. Pertinent descriptive data on the 20 subjects are presented in Table 1. Seven male and 13 female subjects (mean age = 84.65 years) were included. Fifteen percent of subjects scored in the mild range, 50% in the moderate range and 35% in the severe range on the memory cognitive domain of the *CLQT.* Fifteen percent of subjects scored in the mild range, 60% in the moderate range and 25% in the severe range on the language cognitive domain of the *CLQT.* All subjects showed an absence of visual neglect. Subjects' oral reading performance on the reading subtest of the *WRAT-3* ranged from borderline to high average (M = 88.9).

Stimuli

The experimental stimuli consisted of two sets of reading materials: 1) the five generic sentences and pictures from the *BORS* and 2) five equivalent sentences consisting of subject-specific vocabulary and relevant picture supplied by the family. The patient-specific sentences were constructed with the help of family members and corresponding photos were collected. If photos were unavailable clip art was utilized depicting the topic. Table 2 illustrates examples of the generic and subject-specific stimuli. The statements were printed individually on a 5x8 inch horizontal sheet of paper with a 26-point Times New Roman font in black ink. All sheets were placed inside 5x8 inch page protectors and were placed randomly inside a 3-ring binder (5x8 inch), using 1-inch metal rings. The Flesch-Kincaid reading grade level (Kincaid, Aagard, O'Hara, and Cottrell, 1981) was calculated for each of the five personal statements for each subject (20) and for the five generic statements (BORS; Bourgeois, 1992b). This readability measure reports the number of years of U.S. education generally required to understand the written text. The overall mean Flesch-Kincaid reading grade level for personal and generic stimuli was 2.59 (s.d. = 1.36) and 2.60 (s.d. = 2.45) respectively; these means were not significantly different ($t = -.02$; $df = 4$; $p > .05$).

Table 1. Subject Characteristics

Subjects	Sex	Age	CLQT[1] Memory	CLQT Language	Oral Reading[2]	Education
1	M	84	severe	severe	84	High School
2	F	85	severe	moderate	91	10th grade
3	F	81	mild	moderate	81	11th grade
4	F	86	severe	severe	74	High School
5	F	75	moderate	mild	91	High School
6	F	83	moderate	moderate	86	High School
7	F	93	moderate	moderate	95	High School
8	F	84	moderate	moderate	97	9th grade
9	M	91	mild	mild	74	8th grade
10	M	78	severe	severe	66	8th grade
11	F	88	severe	moderate	82	High School
12	F	90	moderate	moderate	86	Some College
13	F	68	severe	moderate	99	Some College
14	F	94	moderate	severe	104	High School
15	F	85	moderate	mild	99	High School
16	F	91	moderate	moderate	95	High School
17	M	83	moderate	moderate	102	Some College
18	M	90	moderate	moderate	99	High School
19	M	85	severe	severe	86	High School
20	M	79	mild	moderate	87	Some College
Mean		84.65			88.9	
SD		6.38			10.22	

Notes: 1. CLQT; Cognitive Linguistic Quick test (Helm-Estabrooks, 2001). 2. WRAT-3; The Wide Range Achievement Test, 3rd ed. (Stone, Jastak, and Wilkinson, 1995) standard score: mean of 100 and a standard deviation of 15.

Data Collection

Each subject participated in two reading sessions within a 7-day period. The experimenter began each 20-minute interaction by shuffling the 10 statement cards to present in a random order and placed the cards inside the 3-ring binder. The presentation order of the cards was tracked on a data sheet for each session. The digital audio recorder (with a timer) was turned on and the prompt "Read this sentence and tell me something about it" was stated. The investigator waited for the subject to read the sentence and to make a comment. If the subject did not make a comment within one minute of reading the sentence, the investigator said, "What do you think about that?" or "Tell me more about this." If the subject was describing the photo instead of talking about the written statement the investigator prompted with, “Tell me more about what this says.” Up to two minutes were allowed for the subject to comment on the reading material.

Table 2. Experimental Stimuli

Generic Stimuli	Sample Personalized Stimuli
The dog’s name is Rover. 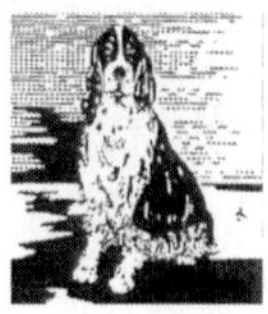	The dog’s name is Rusty. 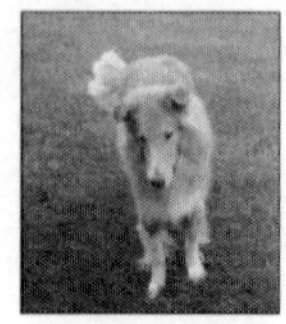
I live in Swissvale. 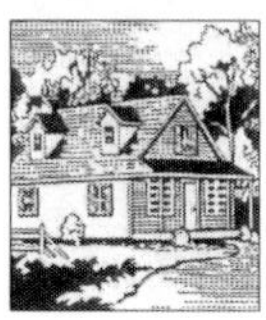	I live in Columbus. 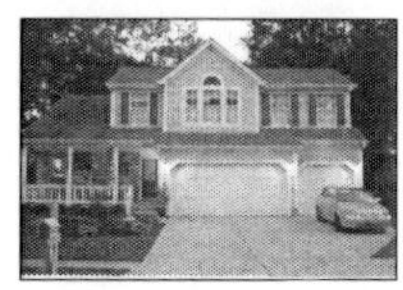
I enjoy baseball games. 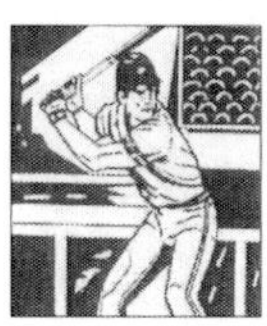	I enjoy reading books. 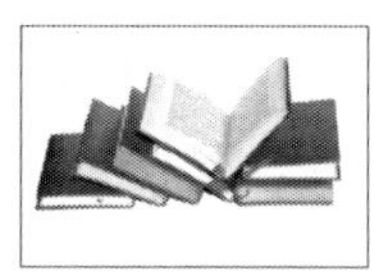
My sister is 75 years old. 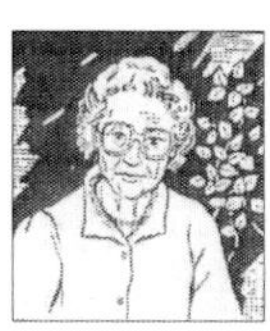	My sister is 96 years old. 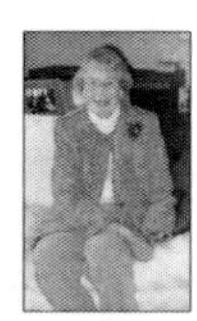
His wife’s name is Mary. 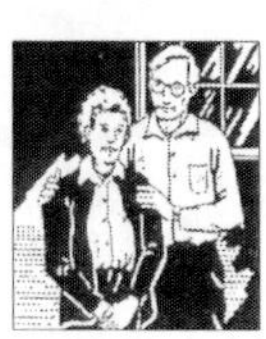	My husband’s name is Harold. 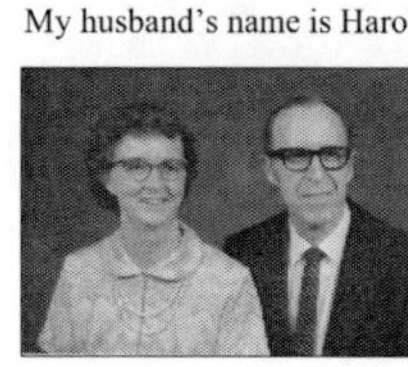

The experimenter listened to the subject’s response, maintained eye contact, and nodded, smiled or made confirming statements to encourage responding. When the subject had finished talking, or after two minutes, the investigator turned the page and stated the prompt to talk about the next statement. For example, “Great, now read this sentence and tell me something about it." Because the prompt did not specify to read aloud or to read silently, if the subject made novel comments based on the written stimuli without reading the sentence aloud, the investigator did not interrupt the subject.

Data Scoring and Analysis

A trained research assistant transcribed all reading sessions from the audio tapes. Each transcript included both subject and investigator utterances. The following dependent variables, adapted from Bourgeois (1990), were coded and summarized for analysis: 1) *Stimulus sentence (percentage of words) read orally (R),* 2) *Novel on-topic statements (N), Comprehension* (*N+) or* (*N-*), and *Photo comment (C),* 3) Additional Utterances: *Ambiguous utterances (A), Repetition of reading (RP), Repetition of information (P), Error statement (E), Other (O), General questions (G), Unintelligible utterances (U),* and 4) Partner utterances: *Investigator prompts (IP), Instructions (I), Investigator other (IO), Investigator filler utterances (IU), Investigator statements (IS), Investigator questions (IQ).* Definitions for each of these dependent variables are included in Table 3.

Table 3. Definitions of Dependent Variables

Stimulus sentence read orally (R)	Percent words read correctly per sentence.
Novel on-topic statements (N)	Intelligible and unambiguous statements or questions contributing additional correct content
I enjoy [baseball games or sport/hobby]	Appropriate pronoun, appropriate referent to the sport or hobby, information about or related to the sport or hobby.
The [dog's or pet's] name is	Appropriate referent to the animal or name, information about or related to the pet. If subject did not own a pet or a photo was unavailable, name of a child or friend was used.
I live in [Swissvale or hometown]	Appropriate referent to place, additional information about or related to Swissvale, the hometown or another city.
His wife's name is [Mary or spouse's name]	Appropriate pronoun, appropriate referent to the spouse or spouse's name, information about or related to the name or the spouse.
My [sister or other relative is 75] years old	Appropriate pronoun, appropriate referent to the person or age, additional information about the indicated person.
Comprehension	
(N+)	Comment that indicates comprehension by addressing the written statement and not describing the picture (e.g. "I live in Swissvale, which I don't know a thing about because I never did live there").
(N-)	Comment that does not indicate comprehension by not directly addressing the written statement (e.g., "come on over Rover").
Photo comment (C)	Intelligible and unambiguous statements related to the picture.
Ambiguous utterances (A)	a) empty phrases (e.g., a common idiom contributing no content to the discourse), b) indefinite terms (e.g., "stuff," "thing," etc.), c) deictic (e.g. "this," "that," "here,") and d) unrelated pronouns or pronouns without antecedents.
Repetition of reading (RP)	Repetition of a previously read stimulus sentence.
Repetition of information (P)	Repetition of previously stated information.

Table 3. (Continued)

Error statement (E)	Intelligible and unambiguous utterances related to the topic sentence that is false, as determined by the experimenter.
Other (O)	Intelligible and unambiguous speech acts such as questions not related to the topic sentence, requests, responses to questions, utterances that regulate the interaction, acknowledgements (e.g. mhmm, yeah, OK, thank you, etc.), commands, social conventions, and unambiguous statements that expressed a fact about topics other than the 10 topic sentences.
General questions (G)	General questions by the investigator or subject unrelated to the topic.
Unintelligible utterances (U)	Laughing; neologisms; literal, verbal, semantic, and phonological paraphasias; sentence fragments; grammatically incomplete sentences; non-English phrases; and multiple joined sentence fragments.
Investigator prompts (IP)	Protocol prompts, "Read this sentence and tell me something about it" and "Tell me more about this."
Instructions (I)	Additional instructive comments related to the activity or the prompt (e.g., read that again, turn the page).
Investigator other (IO)	Acknowledgements of subject utterances and any other utterance to regulate the interaction
Investigator filler utterances (IU)	Laughing; sentence fragments; grammatically incomplete sentences
Investigator statements (IS)	Comments about subject's utterance that provided additional content.
Investigator questions (IQ)	Other requests for information that are not one of the specific prompts. May also be confirmation of information previously stated (e.g. Does he? Not anymore?).

A two-condition (generic vs. personal), within subjects descriptive design with repeated measures (two sessions) was used to compare the effects of two types of reading stimuli on reading comprehension. A paired samples t-test was used to evaluate the differences in the group (generic vs. personal) means for each of the dependent variables.

Reliability

A trained volunteer transcribed all audio recordings of the data collected; the investigator checked the transcriptions against the audio recordings and then coded the behaviors. A second volunteer, trained to a 90% agreement criterion, coded 20% of all the transcripts (8 of 40 total). Percentage of agreement was calculated by dividing the number of agreements by the total number of codes available and multiplying by 100. The inter-observer agreement for all utterances coded was 93% (range 86% to 97%).

Results

Subjects' reading accuracy scores for personal and generic stimuli across the two experimental sessions were compared; a paired samples t-test determined that there was not a significant difference in reading accuracy across data collection sessions with a mean of 91.74

(s.d. = 7.86) for personal stimuli and 94.87 (s.d. = 5.42) for generic stimuli (t = 2.07; df = 19; p > .05). Data for both sessions was averaged for subsequent analysis. Table 4 displays the mean, standard deviation, and p-values of all dependent variables in both experimental conditions.

Table 4. Utterance Analysis s for Personal Stimuli and Generic Stimuli

	Personal		Generic		
Variable	Mean	SD	Mean	SD	P
Oral Reading (Percent)	94.56	6.08	91.67	5.23	*
Novel Responses to Stimuli					
Novel Comment	15.93	7.81	7.3	2.36	***
Comprehension Statement	15.58	8.02	6.73	2.17	***
Non-Comprehension Statement	0.38	0.53	0.58	0.77	NS
Photo Comment	4.03	3.03	3	4.92	NS
Additional Responses to Stimuli					
Ambiguous Utterance	0.08	0.24	0	0	NS
Other	8.55	4.58	4.88	2.36	***
Unintelligible	2.43	1.9	1.43	1.34	**
Error Statement	0.35	0.8	0.08	0.18	NS
Repetition of Reading	1.1	1.22	0.9	1.13	NS
Previously Stated Comment	0.68	0.98	0.2	0.25	*
General Questions	0.05	0.15	0	0	NS
Investigator Utterances					
Investigator Prompts	8.63	2.86	6.5	1.88	***
Additional Instruction	0.98	0.88	0.73	0.73	NS
Investigator Other	13.85	4.75	6.88	2.45	***
Investigator Filler Utterances	0.58	0.57	0.23	0.41	*
Investigator Additional Information	0.73	0.98	0.25	0.55	NS
Investigator Questions	6.88	3.06	3.98	1.7	***

Note. *p < .05, **p < .01, ***p < .001.

The data were grouped into three categories for interpretation: Novel responses to stimuli, Additional responses to stimuli, and Investigator utterances. Figure 1 illustrates the Novel responses to stimuli (total number of novel comments, novel comments indicating reading comprehension, novel comments not indicating reading comprehension and photo comments) averaged across subjects for personal and generic stimuli. As predicted, there were statistically significant differences in the mean number of novel comments for personal (15.93) and generic (7.3) stimuli (t = 5.33; df = 19; p < .001), a large effect (Cohen's *d* = 1.50). Similarly there were significant differences between the means of novel comments reflecting reading comprehension for personal (15.58) and generic (6.73) stimuli (t = 5.23; df = 19; p < .001), a large effect (Cohen's *d* = 1.51). There were no significant differences between means for number of novel comments which did not reflect reading comprehension, nor for number of photo comments.

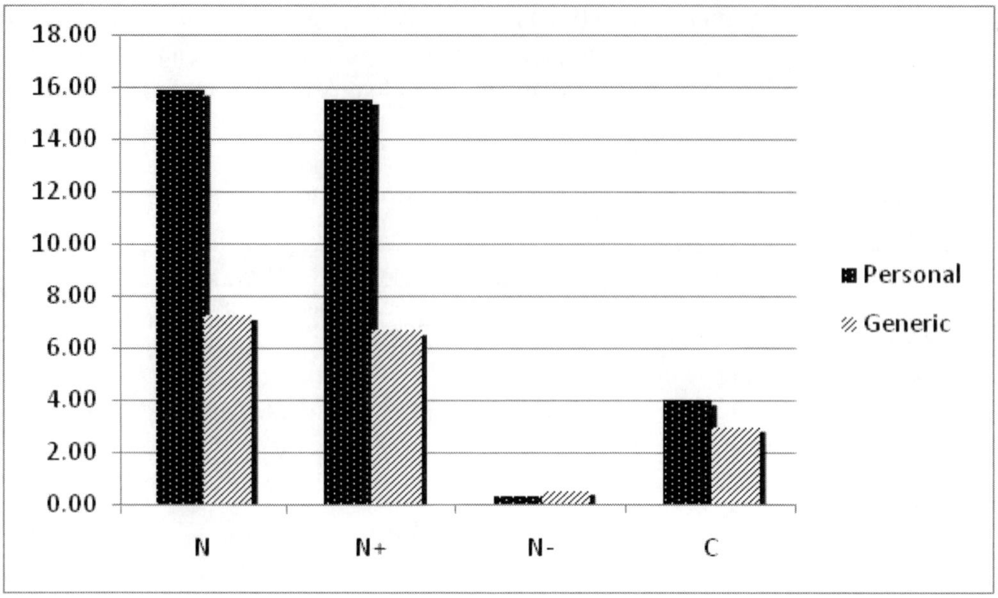

Note: Novel on-topic statements (N), Evidence of Comprehension (N+), No Evidence of Comprehension (N-), Photo comment (C).

Figure 1. Mean Frequencies of Responses to Stimuli by Condition.

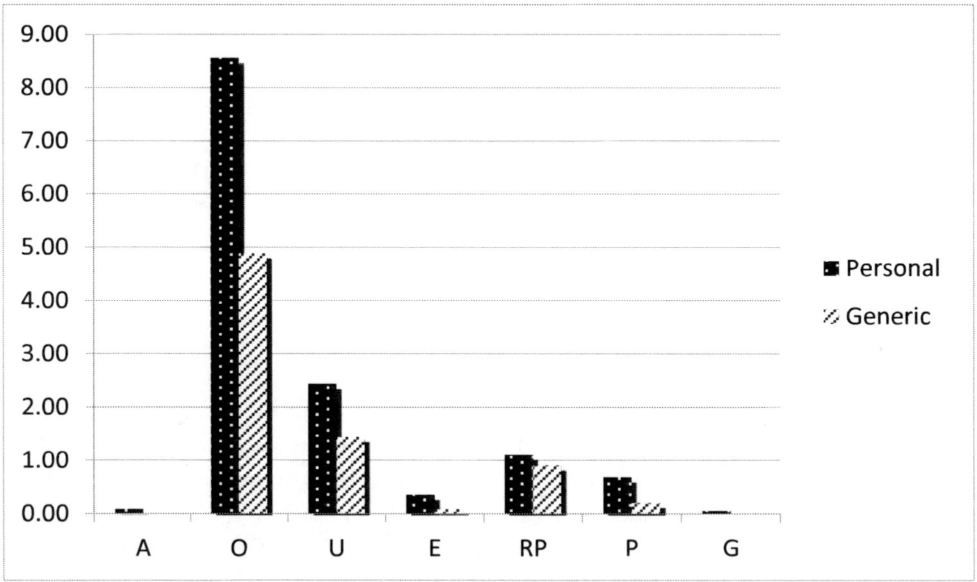

Note: Ambiguous utterances (A), Other (O), Unintelligible utterances (U), Error statement (E), Repetition of reading (RP), Repetition of information (P), General questions (G).

Figure 2. Mean Frequencies of Additional Responses to Stimuli by Condition.

Figure 2 illustrates the Additional responses to stimuli (ambiguous, other, and unintelligible utterances, error statements, repetition of previously read or previously stated information and general questions) for personal and generic stimuli. Statistically significant differences between the means for personal and generic stimuli were found for Other utterances (t = 3.97; df = 19; $p < .001$), Unintelligible utterances (t = 2.79; df = 19; $p < .01$), and Repetitions of previously stated comments (t = 2.37; df = 19; $p < .05$). No differences were found for ambiguous utterances, error statements, repetitions of reading the stimulus, or general questions.

Figure 3 illustrates the Investigator utterances (investigator prompts, additional investigator instructions, investigator other utterances, investigator filler utterances, investigator additional information statements, and investigator questions) for personal and generic stimuli. Statistically significant differences between the means for personal and generic stimuli were found for Investigator prompts (t = 4.42; df = 19; $p < .001$), Investigator other utterances (t = 7.09; df = 19; $p < .001$), Investigator filler utterances (t = 2.21; df = 19; $p < .05$), and Investigator questions (t = 4.05; df = 19; $p < .001$). For all of these dependent variables, the investigator made significantly more utterances in the personal condition. No differences between means were found for Investigator additional instructions or Investigator additional information.

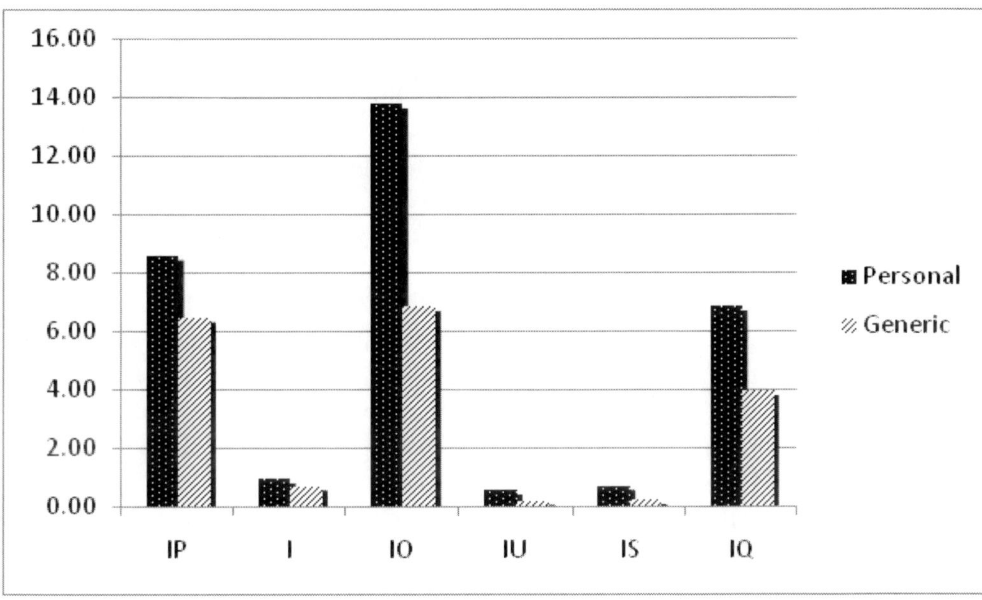

Note: Investigator prompts (IP), Instructions (I), Investigator other (IO), Investigator filler utterances (IU), Investigator statements (IS), Investigator questions (IQ).

Figure 3. Mean Frequencies of Investigator Utterances by Condition.

Conclusion

The purpose of this study was to compare the reading comprehension performance of persons with dementia using generic and personal stimuli. In previous research, reading comprehension was observed in patients with dementia who were asked to read stimuli consisting of generic sentences and pictures (Bourgeois et al., 2002). In contrast, persons with aphasia have been observed to demonstrate better reading comprehension with stimuli including familiar, high-context photographs (Dietz et al., 2009). The results of the current study revealed that personal stimuli produced significantly more novel comments overall and more comments reflecting reading comprehension than generic stimuli. When participants were describing personal stimuli they also produced more other and unintelligible utterances, and they repeated previously stated information more frequently than when describing generic stimuli. This reflects an overall increase in conversational output by the person with dementia when familiar, personal stimuli are used. In addition, more Investigator behaviors, including Investigator prompts, Investigator other, Investigator filler utterances, and Investigator questions, were seen in the personal condition than in the generic condition. It may be that because the subjects were talking more and producing more content in the personal condition, the investigator also talked more, asking a greater number of questions and making more acknowledgements and confirmations. An increased number of prompts were required in the personal condition when the photograph distracted the subject. Some of these utterances were not found to be relevant to the measurement of reading comprehension, so the investigator redirected the subject to the written statement.

In contrast, Novel comments not reflecting comprehension and Photo comments were not significantly different in the personal condition than the generic condition. This supports the assumption that generic photographs and words may not be as effective at helping persons to access relevant memories related to the material. Similarly, Ambiguous utterances, Error statements, and Repetition of reading were not significantly different between the two conditions because subjects appeared to be using these utterances to keep the flow of the conversation going. The fact that there were no differences in the frequency of General questions, Investigator additional instruction, and Investigator additional information across the two conditions confirms that the investigator followed the protocol by limiting her participation in the sessions.

These findings support those of Bourgeois et al. (2002) who found that persons with dementia made novel comments indicative of comprehension after reading generic stimulus sentences. Additionally, the current findings support those of Bourgeois (1990, 1992a, 1993) and Hoerster, Hickey and Bourgeois (2001) who found that memory aids utilizing personal stimuli improved conversational interactions, and were successful in increasing on-topic utterances and decreasing off-topic utterances.

The quantitative and qualitative differences in conversational output for personal and generic stimuli are shown in the following example. When asked to read the generic stimulus, "His wife's name is Mary," one subject stated: "What do you mean about her name is Mary? His wife's name is Mary and she's quite contrary." When shown his personally equivalent stimulus page, he read, "My wife's name is Dorothy." Then he continued, "I call her Dottie and we've been married for 60 years and she's so good. We've had our house for about 40 years and she has taken such good care of it. Not only the house, but around the house, the flowers, the lawn and everything. She just does so well." In the first example the subject was able to read the stimulus sentence with 100% accuracy and knew he was supposed to "say something about it," but was unable to elaborate or express that he did not know the couple shown in the picture. Quite the opposite was demonstrated in the second example where the subject read the sentence with 100% accuracy and then provided ample verbal evidence of comprehension.

An unexpected finding was that there were no statistically significant differences between the numbers of photo comments made in the two conditions; one would have expected more elaborations when viewing personal photos. There were, however, statistically significant differences for Other utterances, Unintelligible utterances and Repetition of previously stated comments made by the subject when viewing personal stimuli suggesting the overall heightened stimulability of the personal stimuli.

The current study confirms the outcomes of the previous studies that reading comprehension can be assessed during an oral reading task with persons with dementia using written and picture stimuli. Furthermore, personal stimuli, reflecting high frequency words and photographs, elicited more verbalizations that can be used to assess reading comprehension performance of persons with dementia than generic stimuli. The fact that persons with dementia demonstrated stability in reading performance over a 7-day period suggests the relative preservation of this cognitive ability. This finding has implications for the use of personal stimuli in other assessment tasks with persons with dementia whose cognitive skills deteriorate over time due to the degenerative nature of their neurological condition.

Future research should extend these findings to a larger, more diverse group of persons with dementia. This study involved a limited number of personal and generic stimuli (five of each); replication of the study with a greater number of generic and personal stimuli for a variety of topics might provide additional insight into what types of stimuli would allow for optimal performance on cognitive assessments. It is important to continue to explore the impact personal stimuli may have on results for the development of evaluation materials to gauge the person's level of functioning and other tools for improving communication. Extending the study to examine the use of personal and generic stimuli in choice making during meal time or other activities of daily living may help to improve the quality of life for persons with dementia and with caregiver interactions. For example, when offering choices of activities, supplementing the choices with pictures of the person with dementia participating in the activities (e.g. reading, watching TV, painting) would be superior to pictures of line drawings. Demonstrating the improved conversational and comprehension abilities of persons with dementia when using personal materials may change the way families and professionals view the abilities of those diagnosed with dementia.

References

Baddeley, A. (1995). The psychology of memory. In A. D. Baddeley, B. A. Wilson, and F. N. Watts (eds.), *Handbook of memory disorders* (pg. 3-26). New York: John Wiley.

Bayles, K. A., and Tomoeda, C. K. (1993). *Arizona battery for communication disorders of dementia*. Phoenix, AZ: Canyonlands.

Bayles, K. A., and Tomoeda, C. K. (1994). *Functional linguistic communication inventory*. Tucson, AZ: Canyonlands.

Bourgeois, M. S. (1990). Enhancing conversation skills in residents with Alzheimer's Disease using a prosthetic memory aid. *Journal of Applied Behavior Analysis, 23*, 29-42.

Bourgeois, M. S. (1992a). Evaluating memory wallets in conversations with persons with dementia. *Journal of Speech and Hearing Research, 35*, 1344-1357.

Bourgeois, M. S. (1992b). *Conversing with memory impaired individuals using memory aids: A memory aid workbook*. Gaylord, MI: Northern Speech Services.

Bourgeois, M. S. (1993). Effects of memory aids on the didactic conversations of individuals with dementia. *Journal of Applied Behavior Analysis, 26*, 77-87.

Bourgeois, M. (2007). *Memory Books and Other Graphic Cuing Systems.* New York: Health Professions Press, Paul H. Brookes Publishing.

Bourgeois, M. S., Dijkstra, K., Burgio, L., and Allen-Burge, R. (November, 1999). Effective communication during care routines: A staff training program. Paper presented at the Gerontological Society of America Conference, San Francisco, CA.

Bourgeois, M. S., Dijkstra, K., Burgio, L., and Allen-Burge, R. (November, 2000). Come talk with me: Improving conversations between residents with dementia and their nursing aides. Symposium paper presented at the Gerontological Society of America, Washington, D.C.

Bourgeois, M. S., and Hickey, E. M. (2009). *Dementia: From diagnosis to management- A functional approach.* New York, NY: Psychological Press.

Bourgeois, M. S., LaPointe, L., Dijkstra, K., Bays, G., Lasker, J., and Johnson, K. (May, 2002). Unexpected evidence of reading comprehension during oral reading in dementia. Presented at the International Clinical Phonetics and Linguistics Association Conference, Hong Kong.

Bourgeois, M. S., and Mason, L. A. (1996). Memory wallet intervention in adult day care setting. *Behavior Interventions: Theory and Practice in Residential and Community-Based Clinical Programs, 11*, 3-18.

Dietz, A., Hux, K., McKelvey, M. L., Beukelman, D. R., and Weissling, K. (2009). Reading comprehension by people with chronic aphasia: A comparison of three levels of visuographic contextual support. *Aphasiology, 23*, 1053-1064.

Helm-Estabrooks, N. (2001). *Cognitive linguistic quick test.* San Antonio, TX: The Psychological Corporation.

Horester, L., Hickey, E. M., and Bourgeois, M.S. (2001). Effects of memory aids on conversations between nursing home residents with dementia and nursing assistants. *Neuropsychological Rehabilitation, 11* (3/4), 399-427.

Kincaid, J. P., Aagard, J. A., O'Hara, J. W., and Cottrell, L. K. (1981). Computer readability editing system. *IEEE Transactions on Professional Communications,* 24 (1), 38-42.

LaPointe, L., and Horner, J. (1998). *Reading comprehension battery for aphasia* (RCBA-2). Austin, TX: Pro-Ed.

Patterson, K., Graham, N., and Hodges, J. (1994). Reading in dementia of the Alzheimer type: A preserved ability? *Neuropsychology, 8*, 395-407.

Stone, M., Jastak, S., and Wilkinson, G. (1995). *Wide Range Achievement Test—3rd Edition.* San Antonio, TX: The Psychological Corporation.

In: Non-Pharmacological Therapies ...
Editor: Elisabetta Farina
ISBN: 978-1-63321-860-4

Chapter 2

Exploring the Use of Two Different Gardens by Residents in a Special Care Unit for People with Dementia

Antonio Guaita, Erminia Gadler, Giovanni Andreoni, Marinella Mancuso, Riccardo Perelli Cippo, Chiara Cutaia, Mauro Colombo and Silvia Vitali
GolgiCenci Foundation and C. Golgi Geriatric Institute, Abbiategrasso, Milan, Italy

Abstract

Backgrounds. The purpose of this study is to examine the use of two different Alzheimer's gardens, one designed as a "quiet space" and the other as an "activity" garden, by direct observations of behavior of the forty two residents in a Special Care Unit for people with dementia.

Methods. Observations were conducted within the gardens to evaluate whether they were used by residents and how, including frequency of visit, way in which the gardens were used for individual and social activities. Since residents are persons with dementia with clinically diagnosed Alzheimer disease, other dementias or psychosis, we compared the recorded behaviors of these three groups.

Results. Findings suggest that the two gardens are used differently in the activities performed according to gender, diagnosis and garden characteristics, while frequency is different only for the time of the day.

Conclusion. These data confirm the importance of the connection between persons with dementia and environment, that can be considered essential part of the therapeutic protocol.

Keywords: Alzheimer disease, dementia, psychosis, therapeutic garden, behavior

Introduction

There is a growing interest in the outdoor spaces and gardens as environments that may be beneficial to the physical health and psychological wellbeing of persons with dementia. Research indicates that access to specially designed gardens is likely to have a general positive influence on patient's behavior, to potentially reduce the number of falls, and to positively affect staff members and the caregivers of the person with dementia (Cohen-Mansfield and Werner 1998, 1999; Detweiler *et al*, 2008; Friedrich, 2009; Heath, 2004; Lawton, 2001; Lee and Kim, 2007; Mooney and Nicell, 1992; Zeisel *et al*, 2003; Zeisel and Tyson, 1999). Nonetheless, the characteristics of the gardens have not been systematically described, therefore it is unclear what are the most advantageous space properties for the person with dementia. Thus, it seems important to understand if different types of outdoor spaces will impact on the behavior and activities of older adults with dementia.

In the larger plan of offering individualized therapeutic environment to people with dementia, two different Alzheimer's ground gardens adjacent to the unit were projected and built. The largest garden, named "Activity Garden," is focused on activities and gardening, and is aimed to decrease apathy providing stimulation with colors, smells, sounds and energetic connection with the environment; while the other, named "Quiet Garden," is focused on lower interaction levels and more restorative functions providing opportunities to relieve tension and aggression, as well as space for reflection and privacy. Both gardens are naturally-mapped environments in the sense that "no instruction book, map or memory is needed to negotiate the environment or figure out how to make the object work…a few clearly recognizable pathways that can be seen from anywhere in the setting, with an entrance and exit that everyone can see and understand as such, and with destinations that users of the environment can see easily" (Zeisel, *Edinburgh Garden Paper*). They have a see-through enclosure and the visibility of both gardens from the inside lies on a continuum.

Both gardens were planned as an important component of the "prosthetic environment", i.e. an adapted physical space needed to avoid stress and danger for the person with dementia derived from an inappropriate demanding environment. The conceptual framework of the "prosthesis" for support people with dementia, better explained elsewhere (Jones, 1999; Colombo *et al*, 2007; Guaita and Jones, 2011), defines essential goals of the physical space not only as safety and security, but also personal comfort and welfare, together with accessibility and flexibility.

Due to safety reasons, the gardens are available at certain times of the day, but during scheduled opening they can be freely used by person with dementia, caregivers, staff and other visitors. Social activities are organized in both gardens. The purpose of this research is threefold: 1) to assess how residents in a Special Care Unit for Dementia actually use and move spontaneously through the outdoor spaces, 2) to determine whether they use the two gardens in different ways, and 3) to gain a more comprehensive understanding of the interaction of person with dementia with environment.

Methods

The research occurred for 3 months (April through July 2010) in a Special Care Unit for Dementia (SPCU). The design framework included time-sampled-observations of the behavior of the all residents and survey of staff and residents' caregivers.

Over this period 229 observational sessions were conducted by two trained research assistants during which a total number of 1031 behaviors were recorded, to analyze behaviors distribution by diagnosis, age, gender, weather conditions, garden, activity performed (detailed map of the gardens in Supplement 1).

Statistical analysis was conducted using Anova, Pearson "r" for linear correlation , student "t-tests" for independent samples and for paired samples when appropriate for parametric variables and square chi for non-parametric variables, using SPSS release 11. Size effect was tested for parametric variables using "r" formula (Rosnow *et al*, 2000).

Residents Assessment

All residents able to move around were recruited in the study (42, including 3 newly admitted), 12 male and 30 female, mean age 80 (±22). Twenty residents have been diagnosed with Alzheimer disease (AD), 16 with dementia (main vascular) (DEM), 6 of them are persons (PSYC) in the late phase of psychosis with cognitive problems after a history of depression and maniac depressive disorders.

The residents were assessed with the following scales:

- Mini-Mental State Examination (MMSE, range 0–30) (Folstein *et* al, 1975): a widely used screening cognitive test, with good reliability and validity;
- Neuro Psychiatric Inventory (NPI, range 0-144) (Cummings *et* al, 1994): the most used checklist of non cognitive symptoms in dementia
- Tinetti Balance (0–16) and Gait (0–12) (Tinetti *et* al, 1986): a performance test to assess the risk of falling in the elderly
- Barthel Index (0–100) (Shah S *et* al, 1989): the most used scale of dependency, weighted in each item.

Observational Protocol

Observation times were scattered throughout the day (10:00, 11:00 and 11:15 am, 1:45, 3:00 and 4:15 pm) in order to record the morning and afternoon activities and to determine when and where the use of gardens occurred. Weather conditions were recorded too and reported as a temperature (Figure 1). To make the observations easier, as well as for safety reasons, one garden was opened, while the other was locked. The sequence of opening was planned to ensure the same availability of both gardens in the morning as well as in the afternoon.

The behavior observation instrument was a paper-and-pencil recording sheet (Supplement 2). To reduce the number of individual variables, either pre-classified or specified by the observers, the recorded activities were reclassified into 6 higher order behavioral categories : rest (sitting alone, dozing, napping); gardening (comprehensive of gardening itself, picking up flowers or fruits, work in the vegetable garden); physical exercise (walking alone or in group, doing exercise); individual engagement (reading, writing, doing paper works, eating, drinking or any activity done by her/himself); spontaneous social activity (chatting, playing cards), engagement in organized activity (group activities proposed by staff such as music-therapy or cognitive stimulation sessions, creative works).

Behavior was recorded noting what each person in the garden was doing during the observation time. Target behaviors were limited to those that could be reliably observed as purposeful, where "purposeful is meant to denote that the act or behavior may be interpreted as directed to the attainment of a goal, i.e. to a final condition in which the behaving object reaches a definite correlation in time or in space with respect to another object or event" (Rosenblueth, Wiener and Bigelow, 1943).

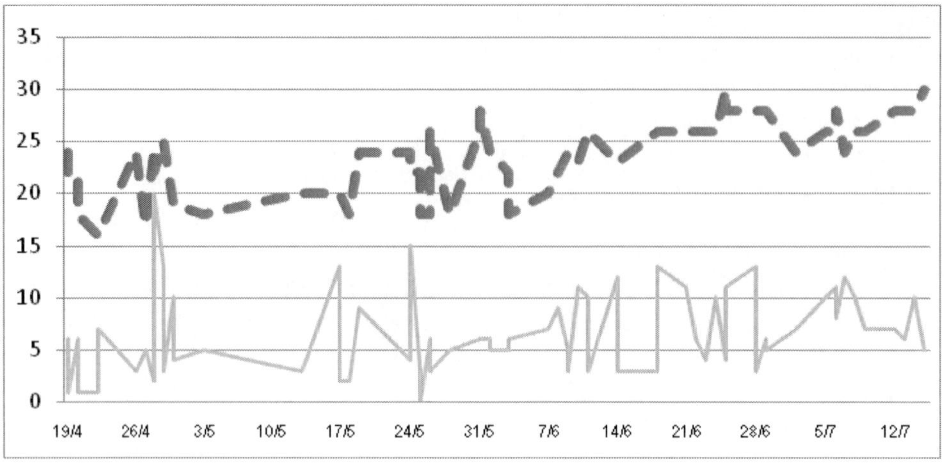

--- = outdoor temperature (C°); — = Number of people. *Not significant correlation.

Figure 1. Frequency of the use of the gardens in relation to weather conditions*.

Modus Operandi

Observations were recorded by two trained research assistants sitting under the gazebos in the gardens. Both assistants were familiar to the residents. They were trained to use checklist and guidelines specifically developed for the study, reaching a good reliability. To prevent observer drift, quality checks of the use of the lists occurred at regular intervals with independent random observations made by a third research assistant who did not routinely collect the data. They assumed the neutral participation approach defined as "a fly on the wall," described for child-watching at playgroup (Sylva *et al*, 1982): they avoided a direct involvement during observation sessions, but did not refuse contact or answers if person with dementia so required.

Observations were performed as one-minute sessions (at 11:00 am and 3:00 pm), and 15-minute sessions (at 10:00 and 11:15 am, at 1:15 and 4:15 pm), during the time that was free of indoor activities for the residents The one minute sessions just recorded "who, where, what" he/she was doing in the garden, and with whom, the kind of activities performed, the number of visitors and/or staff members present in the garden, and the weather conditions.

The 15-min sessions were used to observe 10 target person with dementia [4 persons with Alzheimer Disease (AD), 3 with dementia (DEM), 3 with psychosis (PSYC)], who reflected the mean features and clinical condition of the unit's residents: the research assistants had to record whether target person with dementia were in the garden, to observe what they were performing and any change of activity during the time of observation. If target-person with dementia were not in the garden, the assistant had to wait until the end of the 15-minute session without recording any other patient. The sequence of the target person with dementia to be observed (3 persons per session) was studied in order to ensure an equal number of observations for each group (AD, dementia, psychosis) in both gardens during mornings and afternoons.

The Quiet Garden, was opened less than the Activity Garden due to some maintenance works (27 versus 45 one-minute sessions, with equal distribution between morning and afternoon), so the presences in the two gardens can be compared only using average per session (number of presences divided by number of sessions). Moreover, because this number can be influenced by the different dimension of the considered grouping variable, the mean presence in the garden was also assessed considering all the potential users in the unit (number of presences in the garden divided by number of sessions and by number of persons in the considered category; for example the more numerous female gender can show a higher number of presence per session, but a similar mean presence per person per session compared to the male).

Survey of Staff and Residents' Caregivers

Two different questionnaires were distributed: one to the relatives (one for each resident's family) that were present at list two times a month (29 families out of 42 residents) and one other to all components of the staff (36 subjects), between April and May 2010. 23 caregivers (69 %) and 32 staff members (88,8%) returned the questionnaires.

The two questionnaires shared three main purposes: to explore the perspective of staff and relatives on the gardens used by the person with dementia; to check the feeling of staff and caregivers about the role of the gardens in increasing person with dementia' quality of life; to determine whether the gardens were contributing to the quality of the staff's time.

The 20-items questionnaires were divided into three areas: A) overall importance of the gardens and of each of the possible activities performed outdoor for the wellness of person with dementia, caregivers and staff members (last option only in the staff questionnaire); B) use of the gardens (how often, length of the outdoor visit, alone or with the person with dementia); C) rating of the value of gardens (perceived differences, preferences, evaluations about safety, beauty and harmony, functionality) for person with dementia, caregivers and staff members (last option only in the staff questionnaire).

Setting

The "Activity Garden" is a 3.477 sq. feet ground garden. At the entrance there is a large shadowy veranda with several seats overlooking the whole garden. It offers opportunities for spontaneous encounters and social activities. Two gazebos with seats and benches are available to people looking for private spaces. Several pathways cross the garden. Opposite to the entrance, at the end of the main path, there is a big fountain, and nearby the horticultural area with several plants (vegetables, berries, flowers, fruit trees). This area clearly looks like the typical local horticultural garden. In the Activity Garden, designers have rearranged the plants in order to ensure an active sensory stimulation all year long. Aromatherapy was considered for the selection of herbs and plants, such as bergamot, sage, rosemary, mint, lavender, laurel, basil which are known for their stimulating properties (Price and Price, 1999; Conn and Seitz, 2010; Fujii *et al*, 2008; Lin *et al*, 2007; Bowles *et al*, 2002; Burns, 2002; Holmes *et al*, 2004). The garden is surrounded on two sides by the building of the unit and on the other two sides by a planted green fence.

The "Quiet Garden" is smaller (2.500 sq. feet) and less challenging. It is designed to be a peaceful, safe and enclosed open place. This garden has a main looped pathway, and a seated veranda that allows a view on the lavender isle, on a stone fountain similar to a small cascade, and on the meadows. It is definitely less rich in species: there is only a big bushes of lavender, which has been chosen due to its known quieting properties (Smallwood, 2001; Fujii *et al* 2008; Lin *et al*, 2007; Holmes *et al*, 2002). The south side of the garden offers a seated gazebo and a large cemented area, still waiting to be completed and is less attractive for the person with dementia. It is surrounded on three sides by the buildings of the unit and on the other side by a green fence.

Table 1. Demographic and Mean Values of Clinical Characteristics of Residents of the SPCU

	Gender			Diagnosis			
	Male	emale	*P**	Alzheimer Disease (AD)	Other Dementia (DEM)	Psychotic (PSYC)	*P***
Patients (Number)	12	30	-	20 (16 F)	16 (10 F)	6 (4 F)	-
Age mean (SD)	78 (7,34)	80 (7,99)	*NS*	82 (5,98)	79 (8,1)	73 (8,83)	*<0,05*
Years spent in SPCU mean (SD)	3,36 (3,2)	3,8 (3,6)	*NS*	2,3 (1,9)	3,0 (2,78)	10,6 (8,24)	*<0,05*
MMSE§: mean score (SD)	17,6 (6,34)	13,54 (5,95)	*NS*	12 (3,67)	14,3 (6,92)	18,7 (5,9)	*N.S.*
NPI: mean score (SD)	46,55 (19,61)	42,79 (20,17)	*NS*	37,17 (17,99)	48,27 (20,35)	52,83 (2,27)	*<0,05*
CDR: mean score (SD)	2,36 (1,21)	2,59 (1,03)	*NS*	3,06 (0,24)	2,70 (0,59)	-	*NS*
TINETTI Balance: mean score (SD)	7,91 (4,66)	9,85 (3,82)	*NS*	8,00 (4,47)	9,79 (3,95)	10,20 (4,21)	*N.S.*
TINETTI Gait: mean score (SD)	7,45 (4,03)	9,00 (2,68)	*NS*	7,58 (2,84)	8,93 (3,54)	9,20 (3,49)	*N.S.*
BARTHEL I: mean score (SD)	35,27 (26,57)	32,52 (27,46)	*NS*	21,24 (23,24)	45,60 (23,69)	36,83 (32,87)	*<0,05*

§24 patients could not be evaluated with MMSE due to aphasia or severe cognitive impairment; MMSE = Mini-Mental State Examination; NPI = Neuropsychiatric Inventory; CDR= Clinical Dementia Rating. NS= not significant; * "Student t" ** Anova.

Results

The two groups with dementia (AD and DEM) are homogeneous in terms of age and MMSE at baseline, while the group with a psychiatric history (PSYC) is younger and has been institutionalized for a longer period of time. The clinical stage of the disease is severe and very severe especially for the AD person with dementia, while the non-cognitive problems are more present among the non-AD dementia and psychiatric residents. Barthel Index and Tinetti tests show that low functional level and the gait and balance problems are largely present among the residents. (Table 1).

Frequency of the Use of the Gardens

During the observation period (April through July 2010), 72 one-minute sessions were conducted and 503 occurrences were recorded in the garden. Only once the session was completed with no person with dementia present in the garden, while the average number of residents recorded in the two gardens was 6,99 [SD 4,08]: 7,48 [SD 3,94] in the Quiet Garden and 6,69 [SD 4,13] in the Activity Garden, a non significant difference. Five out of the 42 residents did not use the outdoor space of the gardens. (Table 2). Comparing the frequency of the use of the two gardens by clinical characteristics of the person with dementia, a significant difference was found in the Barthel index (30,33 in the Activity Garden vs. 50,94 in the Quiet Garden; $t = -2{,}364$ $p < {,}05$), while CDR and Tinetti indexes were not significant.

Table 2. Frequency of the use of the gardens*

		Both garden	Activity (ACT)	Quiet (QUI)
Total	Total 1 min session	72	45	27
	Number of presence	503	301	202
	Mean presence/person/session (SD)	0,167 (0,19)	0,159 (0,18)	0,178 (0,21)
	Mean presence/session (SD)	6,99 (4,08)	6,69 (4,13)	7,48 (3,94)

*Not significant differences between the two gardens.

Gender

The gender difference was not statistically significant. The women resulted slightly higher users of the gardens than men (mean access/person/session to the garden: 0,169 [SD 0,16] female vs. 0,159 [SD 0,11] male). Women show only a not significant tendency to prefer the Quiet Garden (mean presence 5,63 [SD 2,76] vs. 4,98 [SD 3,56]), while men are equally present in both gardens. (Table 3).

Table 3. Frequency of the use of the gardens by gender*

		Both garden	Activity (ACT)	Quiet (QUI)
Male	Number of presence (%)	137 (100%)	87 (63,50%)	50 (36,50%)
	Mean presence/person/session (SD)	0,159 (0,11)	0,161 (0,09)	0,154 (0,16)
	Mean presence/session (SD)	3,044 (2,10)	2,29 (1,35)	2,28 (1,32)
Female	Number of presence (%)	366 (100%)	214 (58,47%)	152 (41,53%)
	Mean presence/person/session (SD)	0,169 (0,16)	0,158 (0,15)	0,187 (0,21)
	Mean presence/session (SD)	8,133 (5,23)	4,98 (3,56)	5,63 (2,76)

*Not significant differences in the use of the two gardens by gender.

Morning/Afternoon

On average, person with dementia enter the gardens more frequently in the morning (8,85 [SD 5,63] vs. 5,32 [SD 5,43]). This difference is significant and represents a medium sized effect (t [36]=2,98, p<.005, r=0,45) (Table 4).

Diagnostic Groups

No statistically significant differences were found in the frequency of the use of the gardens among diagnostic groups (table 5).

Table 4. Frequency of use of the gardens during the day*

		Both garden	Activity (ACT)	Quiet (QUI)
Total	Total 1 min session	72	45	27
	Number of session at 11:00	34	21	13
	Number of session at 15:00	38	24	14
11:00	Number of presence (%)	301 (100%)	178 (59,14%)	123 (40,86%)
	Mean presence/person/session (SD)	0,209 (0,17)	0,202 (0,17)	0,22 (0,24)
	Mean presence/session (SD)	8,85 (5,63)	8,48 (4,48)	9,46 (3,41)
15:00	Number of presence (%)	202 (100%)	120 (59,40%)	82 (40,60%)
	Mean presence/person/session (SD)	0,170 (0,18)	0,122 (0,16)	0,14 (0,19)
	Mean presence/session (SD)	5,32 (5,43)	5,0 (2,81)	6,30 (2,96)

* Both gardens are more frequented in the late morning; the difference is significant (p< ,005).

Table 5. Frequency of the use of the gardens by diagnostic group*

		Both garden	Activity (ACT)	Quiet (QUI)
Total	Total 1 min session	72	45	27
AD	Number of presence (%)	164 (100%)	115 (70,12%)	49 (29,88%)
	Mean presence/person/session (SD)	0,114 (0,10)	0,128 (0,10)	0,09 (0,12)
	Mean presence/session (SD)	4,49 (1,89)	2,56 (4,48)	1,81 (3,41)
DEM	Number of presence (%)	230 (100%)	122 (53,04%)	108 (46,96%)
	Mean presence/person/session (SD)	0,2 (0,26)	0,169 (0,16)	0,25 (0,22)
	Mean presence/session (SD)	6,30 (1,89)	2,71 (1,73)	4,0 (1,90)
PSYC	Number of presence (%)	109 (100%)	64 (58,71%)	45 (41,29%)
	Mean presence/person/session (SD)	0,252 (0,15)	0,237 (0,13)	0,28 (0,21)
	Mean presence/session (SD)	2,99 (1,06)	1,42 (1,05)	1,67 (1,07)

*Not significant differences between the two gardens by diagnostic groups.

The presence of AD residents is positively related to the number of people co-present in the garden (Table 6), while this correlation is negative for other people with dementia (r=-.977, p<.01) (Figure 2). No relationship was found for psychotic person.

Table 6. % of patients in the gardens by diagnosis and number of co-presences

	Patients in the outdoor gardens:		
Co-presence of residents in the gardens	AD (47,6%)	DEM (38,1%)	PSYC (14,3%)
1-2 pp.	12%	63%	25%
3-5 pp.	20%	53%	27%
6-9 pp.	25%	49%	26%
10-13 pp.	34%	47%	19%
14+ pp.	47%	32%	21%

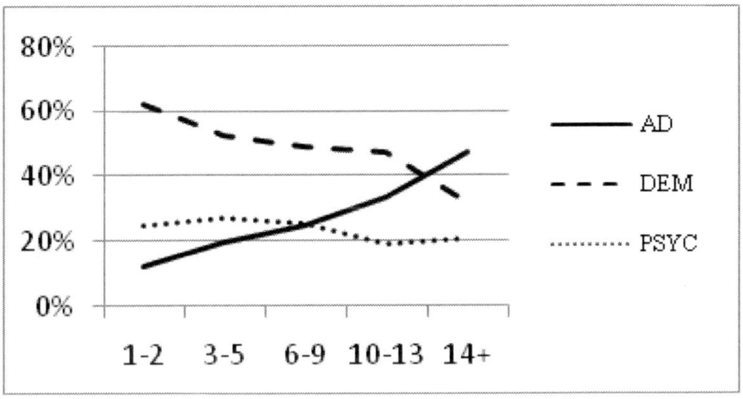

*The number of AD patients increases in the gardens when other persons are present, while the number of DEM decreases (p < 0,01; Spearman "r" linear correlation). No correlation for the PSYC patients.

Figure 2. Correlations between co-presences and diagnostic groups*.

Outdoor Activity

Activity Difference in the Two Gardens

The activities performed outdoor are mainly social (50,3%), either organized by the staff (40%) or by spontaneous engagement of the person with dementia. Rest is a relevant and frequent activity (34,6%), while gardening does hardly attract person with dementia (7%) despite the support of a dedicated volunteer. Physical activity and individual engagement are much less frequent than social activities or rest. The type of activities performed does not significantly differ between the two gardens (Table 7).

Gender Differences

There are significant differences in the performed activities by gender (χ^2= 15,149, p< ,01). Women are more inclined in resting and spontaneous social engagement, while male are more present in physical exercise, individual engagement, organized social activity. (Table 8).

Table 7. Activities performed outdoor*

Behaviour in the gardens	Total	Rest			Gardening		Physical Exercise		Individual Engagement		Social Engagement (organized)		Social (spontaneous)	
	ACT	QUI	ACT	QUI	ACT	QUI	ACT	QUI	ACT	QUI	ACT	QUI	ACT	QUI
Percentage	100%	100 %	34,9%	34,2%	1,7%	1%	7%	8,4%	5,3%	6,9%	39,9%	39,6%	11,2%	9,9%
Count	301	202	105	69	5	2	21	17	16	14	120	80	34	20

ACT= "Activity Garden"; QUI="Quiet Garden"
*Not significant differences between the two gardens in the total number of activities.

Table 8. Gender difference in the activities in the gardens*

activities in the gardens	Total		Rest		Gardening		Physical Exercise		Individual Engagement		Social Engagement (organized)		Social (spontaneous)	
	FEMALE	MALE	FEMALE	MALE	FEMALE	MALE	FEMALE	MALE	FEMALE	MALE	FEMALE	MALE	FEMALE	MALE
Percentage	100%	100%	37,7%	26,3%	1,6%	0,7%	5,7%	12,4%	4,6%	9,5%	38,8%	42,3%	11,6%	8,8%
Count	366	137	138	36	6	1	21	17	17	13	142	58	42	12

*Male and female have different distribution in the type of activities , in the two gardens (more rest for female and more physical exercise for male)(p< 0,01).

Table 9. Difference between diagnostic groups*

	Total of Behavior		Rest		Gardening		Physical Exercise		Individual Engagement		Social Engagement (organized)		Social (spontaneous)	
DIAGNOSIS	ACT	QUI	ACT	QUI	ACT	QUI	ACT	QUI	ACT	QUI	ACT	QUI	ACT	QUI
AD	115	49	40,9%	34,7%	0,0%	0,0%	9,6%	12,2%	2,6%	2,0%	35,6%	42,9%	11,3%	8,2%
DEM	122	108	32,8%	29,6%	3,3%	1,8%	6,6%	10,2%	5,7%	8,3%	40,2%	37,9%	11,4%	12%
PSYC	64	45	28,1%	44,4%	1,6%	0,0%	3,1%	0,0%	9,4%	8,9%	46,9%	40,0%	10,9%	6,7%
Total	301	202	105	69	5	2	21	17	16	14	120	80	34	20

ACT= "Activity Garden"; QUI="Quiet Garden".
* Different distribution of the activities in the two gardens, according to diagnostic groups (p< ,003).

Diagnostic Groups

There are significant differences in the activities performed in the two gardens by diagnosis (χ^2= 11,693, p< ,003). Persons with dementia show a tendency to prefer the Activity Garden for resting and the Quiet Garden for social organized activities, on the contrary psychotics seem to prefer the Quiet Garden for resting and the Activity Garden for social organized activities (Table 9).

Change of Activities Recorded during the Prolonged 15-Min-Sessions

During the 15-min-sessions all transition of states and the behavior state following each transition by 10 target person with dementia of the unit were recorded. 336 presences in the garden were observed.

Most of the time (57,9%) person with dementia did not change their activity during the observational session. Continuity was more frequent during the morning (66% vs. 45,3% in the afternoon), among women (36,5% vs. 23,8%) and depending on the garden. In the Quiet Garden, 64,1% of the observations recorded one single activity per patient (vs. 41,3% in the Activity Garden) and 14,6% one change of state (vs. 21,1% in the other garden) (Table 10).

Table 10. Change of activities in the two gardens

Number of changes in the activities performed	ACT	QUI
0	41,3%	64,1%
1	21,1%	14,6%
2	11,9%	15,5%
3	7,3%	4,9%
4	0,0%	1,0%

ACT= "Activity Garden"; QUI="Quiet Garden".

Survey of Relatives and Staff

Of the 65 questionnaires distributed , 29 to relatives and 36 to staff members, 55 persons returned the questionnaire (84,6%). 91,3% of caregivers and 100% of staff members say that gardens have a positive influence on person with dementia (9,7% of caregivers answered that they didn't know). According to 78,3% of caregivers and 96,9% of staff members it is preferable to spend time with the person with dementia in the garden rather than inside the building, since 87% of caregivers and 93,8% of staff members feel better (i.e., more relaxed, less thoughtful, happier) after a visit outside, and they believe that also person with dementia feel better (more relaxed, smiling, feeling like home). None of the caregivers or staff members said that person with dementia seemed to feel worse after having spent time in the gardens.

Table 11. Caregivers and staff members garden preference and residents' rated preference*

	Preference			Opinion about Residents' Preference			
	ACT	QUI	DON'T KNOW	ACT	QUI	DON'T KNOW	UNABLE TO DISTINGUISH
Caregivers	39,10%	21,70%	39,10%	8,7%	8,7%	52,20%	30,40%
Staff	59,40%	21,90%	18,70%	25%	6,30%	40,30%	28,10%

ACT= "Activity Garden"; QUI="Quiet Garden".

* note that both caregivers and staff prefer ACT garden, but there is a high percentage that does not have an opinion; the same is reported about the residents ability to make.

39,1% of caregivers and 18,7% of staff members said that they did not see or could tell the difference between the two gardens. The Activity Garden is preferred by 39,1% of the caregivers and 59,4% of staff, while the Quiet Garden by 21,7% of caregivers and 21,9% of staff . Only 8,7% of the caregivers rated that person with dementia felt difference between the gardens, although 52,2% of them stated to ignore the real preference of the residents and 30,4% felt that residents could not tell the difference. Residents prefer the Activity Garden, according to 25% of the staff members and the Quiet Garden according to 6,3% of them, but 40,3% acknowledged to ignore the residents' preference and 28,1% believed they cannot tell the difference (Table 11).

Discussion

The two gardens were frequented by a large number of residents, so we can say that outdoor space is a component of the living space they willingly use. The feature of the unit could have favored it, as the gardens are fully visible from the large windows and glass doors of the corridors.

The outdoor space resulted in a frequented and welcome space, where the residents could display different choices.In fact they showed to prefer the morning that is in general the period of the day they have more energy (Jones, 1999; Cohen Mansfield, 2007) and the gardens have better lighting and a comfortable temperature. The residents also showed a broad range of activities during the time they spent outdoor, from a quiet looking at a beautiful space sitting on a chair to an active gardening. It is true that the majority of the time was spent, more often in the Quiet Garden, in performing a single activity rather than experiencing different occupations, but this is expected in a cognitive impaired population where any change is extremely costly in terms of personal energy (Jones, 1999).

The data indicate that the two gardens are perceived and used differently based on specific characteristics of the residents, mainly gender and diagnosis. The Activity Garden is frequented more than the Quiet Garden by the residents with less ability. This unexpected result comes mainly from the preference of the persons with AD, that are more dependent and more present in the Activity Garden. The preference of the AD person with dementia for the Activity Garden may have different explanations, based on the shape of the garden as well as on the features of the person with AD. It is well known that AD modifies vision function precociously, so to alter contrast sensitivity and 3D distance evaluation (Kavcic *et al*, 2006), with a longer time of adaptation to a different lighting intensity (Neargarder *et al*, 2003). The Activity Garden had more plants and fences so the empty spaces may be smaller and the more pronounced color contrasts make easier to see the details. Moreover the presence of other persons in the gardens seems to favor the presence of the AD persons. Women seemed to prefer more relaxing and contemplative interaction with the outdoor environment, while men were more often engaged in active tasks. This agree with the non significant tendency of the women to stay in the Quiet Garden but the data do not allow a conclusive consideration about this aspect of gender difference; furthermore very little is known in general about gender diversity in individuals with dementia (Ott *et al*, 1996). Gardening, not surprisingly, was less practiced by these persons, that are in a severe and very severe stage of the disease, when executive functions are deeply impaired.

Staff and relatives show some similarities and some differences in their evaluations of the meaning of the gardens. The differences between gardens were less evident for the staff than for the relatives, though both preferred the Activity Garden. The ability to choose the preferred garden by the residents was underestimated by relatives and staff. They did not ask the patient's preferences and believed the residents were unable to express a choice. Finally they shared a large positive impression about the presence of the gardens, both for the person with dementia and for themselves.

Conclusion

Despite some limitations (not a case control study, evident impracticality to blind the raters, different numbers of observations on the two gardens, gardens not opened simultaneously) this is the first study that uses direct observations to evaluate the use of two differently designed gardens by residents with dementia. Our data suggest that the activities rather than the frequency of use were influenced by the different design of the two gardens. The main purpose of the study was to assess how different outdoor spaces can be perceived by residents, relatives and staff and potentially influence the behavior in term of activities, so no conclusions can be drawn about the influence of the gardens on the general well being of the residents.

More studies need to be conducted for testing the effect of different designed outdoor spaces on the behavior problems and the need of assistance of people with dementia resident in a special care unit.

References

Bowles, E. J., Griffiths, D. M., Quirk, L., *et* al (2002) Effects of essential oils and touch on resistance to nursing care procedures and other dementia related behaviours in a residential care facility. *International Journal of Aromatherapy*. 12, 22–29.

Burns, A., Byrne, J., Ballard, C., *et* al (2002) Sensory stimulation in dementia. An effective option for managing behavioural problems. *British Medical Journal*. 325, 1312–1313.

Cohen-Mansfield J. (2007) Temporal patterns of agitation in dementia. *American Journal of Geriatric Psychiatry*. 15, 395–405.

Cohen-Mansfield J., Werner P. (1999) Outdoor wandering parks for persons with dementia: a survey of characteristics and use. *Alzheimer Disease and Associated Disorders*. 13, 109–117.

Cohen-Mansfield, J., Werner, P. (1998) The effects of an enhanced environment on nursing home residents who pace. *The Gerontologist*. 38, 199-208.

Colombo M, Vitali S, Cairati M, Vaccaro R, Andreoni G, Guaita A. (2007) Behavioural and psychotic symptoms of dementia (BPSD) improvements in a special care unit: a factor analysis. *Archives of Gerontology and Geriatrics*. 44, 113-120.

Conn D.K., Seitz D.P. (2010) Advances in the treatment of psychiatric disorders in long-term care homes. *Current Opinion in Psychiatry*. 23, 516-521.

Cooper Marcus C., Barnes. M. (1995). *Gardens in Health Care Facilities: Uses, Therapeutic Benefits, and Design Considerations*. Martinez, CA: The Center of Health Design.

Cooper Marcus C., Barnes. M. (Eds.) (1999) *Healing Gardens: Therapeutic Benefits and Design Recommendations*. New York: John Wiley and Sons.

Cummings JL, Mega M, Gray K, Rosenberg-Thompson S, Carusi DA, Gornbein J. (1994) The Neuro-psychiatric Inventory: comprehensive assessment of psychopathology in dementia. *Neurology*. 44, 2308–2314.

Detweiler M.K., Murphy P.F., Myers L.C., Kim K.Y. (2008) Does a wander garden influence inappropriate behaviors in dementia residents? *American Journal of Alzheimer's Disease and Other Dementias*. 23, 31-45.

Folstein M.F., Folstein S.E., McHugh P.R. (1975) Mini-mental state: A practical method for grading the cognitive state of patients for the clinician. *Journal of Psychiatric Research*. 12, 189-198.

Friedrich M.J. (2009) Therapeutic Environmental Design Aims to Help Patients With Alzheimer Disease, *JAMA*. 301, 2430.

Fujii M., Hatakeyama R., Fukuoka Y., Yamamoto T., Sasaki R., Moriya M., Kanno M., Sasaki H. (2008) Lavender aroma therapy for behavioral and psychological symptoms in dementia patients. *Geriatrics and Gerontology International*. 8, 136-138.

Guaita A., Jones M. (2011) A "Prosthetic" Approach for Individuals With Dementia? *JAMA*. 305, 402-403.

Heath Y. (2004) Evaluating the effect of therapeutic gardens. *American Journal of Alzheimer's Disease and Other Dementias*. 19, 239-242.

Holmes C, Hopkins V, Hensford C, MacLaughlin V, Wilkinson D, Rosenvinge H. (2002) Lavender oil as a treatment for agitated behaviour in severe dementia: a placebo controlled study. *International Journal of Geriatric Psychiatry*. 17, 305-308.

Holmes C., Ballard C. (2004) Aromatherapy in dementia. *Advances in Psychiatric Treatment*. 10, 296-300.

Hughes C. P., Berg L., Danziger W. L., *et* al (1982) A new clinical scale for the staging of dementia. *British Journal of Psychiatry*. 140, 566-572.

Jones M. (1999) *GentleCare: Changing the Experience of Alzheimer's Disease in a Positive Way*. Vancouver, British Columbia, Canada: Hartley and Marks Publishers.

Kavcic V., Fernandez R., Logan D., Duffy C.J. (2006) Neurophysiological and perceptual correlates of navigational impairment in Alzheimer's disease. *Brain*. 129, 736-746.

Lawton M. P. (2001) The physical environment of the person with Alzheimer's disease. *Aging and Mental Health*. 5, Supplement 1, S56-64.

Lee Y., Kim S. (2007) Effects of indoor gardening on sleep, agitation and cognition in dementia patients-a pilot study. *International Journal of Geriatric Psychiatry*. 23, 485-489.

Lin P.W., Chan W.C., Ng B.F., Lam L.C. (2007) Efficacy of aromatherapy (Lavandula angustifolia) as an intervention for agitated behaviours in Chinese older persons with dementia: a cross-over randomized trial. *International Journal of Geriatric Psychiatry*. 22, 405-410.

Mooney P., Nicell P.L. (1992) The importance of exterior environment for Alzheimer residents: Effective care and risk management. *Healthcare Management Forum*. 5, 23-29.

Neargarder S.A., Stone E.R., Cronin-Golomb A., Oross S. (2003) The impact of acuity on performance of four clinical measures of contrast sensitivity in Alzheimer's disease. *The Journals of Gerontology Series B*. 58, 54-62.

O'Connor D.W., Ames D., Gardner B., King M. (2009) Psycho-social treatments of behavior symptoms in dementia: a systematic review of reports meeting quality standards. *International Psychogeriatrics*.21, 225-240.

Ott B.R., Tate C.A., Gordon N.M., Heindel W.C. (1996) Gender differences in the behavioral manifestations of Alzheimer's disease. *Journal of the American Geriatrics Society*. 44, 583-587.

Price S., Price L. (1999) *Aromatherapy for Health Professionals*. London: Churchill Livingstone.

Rosenblueth A., Wiener N., Bigelow J. (1943) Behavior, Purpose and Teleology. *Philosophy of Science*. 10, 18-24.

Rosnow P.L, Rosenthal R., Rubin D.B. (2000). Contrasts and correlations in effect-size estimation. *Psychological Science*. 11, 446-453.

Shah S, Vanclay F, Cooper B. (1989) Improving the sensitivity of the Barthel Index for stroke rehabilitation. *J Clin Epidemiol.;* 42, 703-9.

Smallwood J., Brown R., Coulter F., *et* al (2001) Aromatherapy and behaviour disturbances in dementia: a randomized controlled trial. *International Journal of Geriatric Psychiatry*. 16, 1010–1013.

Sylva K., Roy C, Painter M (1982) *Childwatching at Playgroup and Nursery School*, London: Grant McIntyre.

Tinetti M.E., Williams T.F., Mayewski R. (1986) Fall risk index for elderly patients based on number of chronic disabilities. *American Journal of Medicine*. 80, 429-434.

Zeisel J., Tyson M. (1999) Alzheimer's treatment gardens. In: Cooper Marcus C. and Barnes M. (eds.), *Healing Gardens: Therapeutic Benefits and Design Recommendations*. John Wiley and Sons.

Zeisel J. Treatment Effects of Healing Gardens for Alzheimer's: A Difficult Thing to Prove, *Edinburgh Garden Paper*. www.openspace.eca.ac.uk/conference/proceedings/PDF /Zeisel.pd.

Zeisel J., Silverstein N., Hyde J., Levkoff S., Lawton M.P., Holmes W. (2003) Environmental correlates to behavioral outcomes in Alzheimer's special care units. *The Gerontologist*. 43, 697-711.

In: Non-Pharmacological Therapies ...
Editor: Elisabetta Farina

ISBN: 978-1-63321-860-4

Chapter 3

Practical Protocol for Implementing Cognitive Stimulation in Persons with Delirium Superimposed on Dementia

***Ann M. Kolanowski*[1*], *Nikki Hill*[1], *Linda Clare*[2] and *Patricia Marx*[1]**
[1]School of Nursing, Pennsylvania State University, University Park, PA, US
[2]Department of Psychology, Bangor University, Wales, UK

Abstract

Delirium is common in persons with dementia and often accompanies acute medical or surgical conditions. These individuals are at risk for an accelerated decline in their cognitive and physical function. For this reason, interventions that help resolve delirium are critically needed. We have developed a non-pharmacological intervention for delirium in persons with dementia based on our prior interdisciplinary work on delirium, dementia and cognitive stimulation. The intervention uses recreational activities that are alerting, capture attention, and provide cognitive stimulation that encourages cognitive processing in support of cognitive function. In this paper we describe the practical protocol we have developed for implementing these activities, and present a video that will enhance treatment fidelity for studies that replicate the approach.

Keywords: Cognitive stimulation, recreational activities, delirium, dementia

Introduction

Delirium is defined as a state of increased confusion that is a change from a prior level of functioning and is characterized by a fluctuating decline in cognitive function [1]. Inattention

* Corresponding author: E-mail address: amk20@psu.edu, Telephone: 814-863-990, Fax: 814-865-3779

is the primary neuropsychological deficit in delirium. It is not known what causes change in cognition, but delirium is often observed following an insult such as surgery, infection, or adverse medication effects [2]. Delirium is prevalent and deadly in older adults with dementia, those at highest risk. An overwhelming majority of persons with dementia experience delirium when hospitalized, and studies report that between 24 and 76% die within one year of the index episode [3, 4]. It is not uncommon for delirium to persist for months in survivors. These individuals are at risk for an accelerated decline in their cognitive and physical function. Prevention is always a priority; however, it is often difficult to *prevent* delirium in this population because of their already reduced cognitive reserve. For this reason, interventions that help resolve delirium are critically needed. Unfortunately, there are few interventions that treat established delirium at the current time because its etiology is not completely understood.

Our research team has developed a non-pharmacological intervention for delirium in persons with dementia based on over 15 years of research and clinical experience. Non-pharmacological approaches are especially desirable in persons with delirium and dementia because many of the medications used in treatment of this syndrome may actually precipitate delirium and contribute to further long term cognitive impairment [5, 6]. Briefly, the intervention uses recreational activities that are alerting, capture attention, provide cognitive stimulation, and thereby encourage cognitive processing in order to support cognitive function.

The study that will test the efficacy of our protocol has been funded by the National Institute of Nursing Research (R01 NR012242), and has received approval from the Pennsylvania State University Institutional Review Board (IRB# 33443). The underlying theory supporting the intervention [7] and the full study protocol [8] have been published. This paper supplements those prior papers by describing, in detail, the *practical* protocol we have developed for implementing cognitive stimulation using simple recreational activities as the vehicle for delivery. A video that illustrates implementation of the intervention accompanies this paper. Our goal is to distribute the practical protocol to a wide audience so that it can be replicated and tested in other settings.

Background

The pathophysiology of delirium has been described and represents a transient disruption of cerebral homeostasis including disruption of cholinergic transmission, dopaminergic excess and inflammation [2]. Clinically there is inattention (the primary neuropsychological deficit), an altered level of consciousness that can range from stupor to hyperviglience, and disorganized thinking. Because the attentional system is a key mechanism in this syndrome, interventions that support attentional skills, which are necessary for cognitive processing in other domains, may assist in recovery from delirium. In addition to attention, we target other cognitive domains affected by delirium: orientation, memory, abstract thinking and executive function.

Cognitive stimulation is a non-regimented intervention that promotes cognitive processing in order to restore cognitive function [9]. Many activities provide cognitive stimulation. Recreational activities such as word searches, board games, or card games deliver cognitive stimulation in a very unobtrusive, enjoyable manner making them particularly appropriate for individuals who may not tolerate formal methods of cognitive training [10]. In our protocol, we use recreational activities that are tailored to personal interests and functional abilities. Attributes of personal interests are that they focus attention, arouse feelings and promote engagement [11]. Research has also shown that when an individual's functional skills are equal to the challenges inherent in an activity, the individual is more likely to become fully engaged, lose track of time, and experience positive emotions [12] Activities that are personally interesting and designed to accommodate functional skills provide intrinsic motivation for participation and help to ensure long term participation, a requisite for maximum benefit [13]. In clinical trials and other studies our tailored activities have repeatedly demonstrated the ability to alert, to increase attention and to engage persons with dementia compared to non-tailored activities [14- 16].

Procedure

The following is a description of our practical protocol for implementing cognitively stimulating recreational activities in our current study which takes place in post-acute care settings. To tailor recreational activities so they support cognitive processing, we begin by obtaining data on each study participant's cognitive function, physical function, and activity interests. Standardized instruments with known reliability are used. A research nurse conducts the cognitive and physical function assessments and a close family member provides information on activity interests. In our work we use the Modified Blessed Dementia Rating Scale [17], the Clinical Dementia Rating Scale [18], and the Mini-mental State Exam [19] to assess cognitive function; the Barthel Index [20] to assess physical function; and an adapted version of the Farrington Interest Inventory [21] to assess activity interests. Specific cognitive deficits are noted so that activities are selected to be sufficiently, but not overly, challenging. If spacial orientation is a problem, for example, it might be best to initially avoid puzzles. Many activities depend on vision and /or hearing; for participants with sensory impairments, adjustments need to be made. For example, a hearing amplifier may assist individuals with hearing loss. For participants with vision loss, activities that rely primarily on hearing can be substituted.

Based on the assessment, tailored recreational activities designed around themes of interest are selected by level of difficulty (easy, moderate, and difficult) in the cognitive domains of attention, orientation, memory, abstract thinking and executive functioning. Table 1 lists examples of these activities. As an illustration, an older woman who is in a mild stage of dementia with no severe sensory impairments and whose prior interests involved baking, sewing and gardening might be prescribed: identify the sound of a sewing machine (attention); discuss whether the current calendar month is good for planting (orientation); use memory tray with three or more baking utensils (memory); describe steps to prepare a meal (abstract thinking); and work an "activity apron" (executive functioning).

Activities are implemented for 30 minutes each day, a dosage recommended by expert recreational therapists from the American Therapeutic Recreation Association and the National Recreation Society [22], standard recreational therapy practice in the nursing home, and studies that have demonstrated the efficacy of daily, 30-minute recreational therapy for behavioral symptoms and functional impairment in persons with dementia [23-25].

Table 1. Activities by Cognitive Domain and Level of Difficulty

ATTENTION
EASY
Recite the alphabet to the letter "L"
MODERATE
Dot to Dot: connect numbers or letters in sequence
DIFFICULT
Find the Differences: show two similar pictures and identify the difference
ORIENTATION
EASY
Game of "Where am I?" Describe general places (Big city, the beach etc. Example: I am in a place that has tall buildings, a lot of traffic and noise. Where am I? (Big City)
MODERATE
Calendar work: have participant identify month selected, how many days, weeks, holidays in the month
DIFFICULT
Discuss current events from Newspaper
MEMORY
EASY
"Finish the Phrase" cards- use well known phrases. Ex: begin the phrase " A stitch in time" … allow the participant finish the phrase.. " saves nine"
MODERATE
Identify famous faces (movie stars, historical figures from pictures and books)
DIFFICULT
"Memory Tray"- show a tray of 5 items familiar to the participant for one minute. Ask participant to write down as many as possible from memory
ABSTRACT THINKING
EASY
Fanfare cards- pick a category & have participant turn over each card & see if it belongs in the category- if it does, keep face up- if not return face down on table.
MODERATE
Challenge List: Things that can Fly, Things that are invisible… Ex: Ask participant to name 3 things that can fly [a bird, a plane, a bee]. Name 3 girls names, 3 tools or kitchen gadgets etc.
DIFFICULT
"Price is Right" game- Ask participant to arrange items (food, tools, etc.) in order of price. Ex: Place a box of noodles, a jar of Peanut Butter and a can of Coffee in front of the participant. Ask participant to put the items in order from lowest price to highest.
EXECUTIVE FUNCTIONING
EASY
Sort items by color/shape. Use foam or wood block shapes
MODERATE
Calculate change for a purchase
DIFFICULT
Game of "Hangman"

There are several approaches that help maximize the benefits study participants receive from their prescribed cognitive activities. While the activities themselves are simple and easy to implement, they take considerable planning and organization to ensure treatment fidelity. Our procedure is based on guidance from the literature and over 15 years of experience in the field.

Activity Resources

1. Buettner L, Martin SL: *Therapeutic recreation in the nursing home*. State College, PA: Venture Pub. 1995.
2. Buettner LL: Simple Pleasures: A multilevel sensorimotor intervention for nursing home residents with dementia. *American Journal of Alzheimer's Disease and Other Dementias* 1999, 14(1):41-52.
3. Fitzsimmons, S: *Brain Fitness: An instructor's manual of 154 exercises for persons with low to high cognitive function.* Venture Publishing, State College, Pa. 2008
4. Kolanowski A, Buettner L, Fick D, Fitzsimmons S, Cornacchione M: Instituting cognitive rehabilitation in post-acute care. *Annals of Long-Term Care.* 2008;16(2) :40-46.
5. Spector A, Thorgrimsen L, Woods B, Orrell M: *Making a difference: An evidence-based programme to offer cognitive stimulation therapy (CST) to people with dementia*. London: Hawker Publications. 2006.

Both the participant and the environment should be prepared for implementation of the intervention. During the intervention, use of proper communication techniques with participants who have delirium and dementia is vital to implementation. We also incorporate principles for implementing cognitive activities as outlined by Green and Bavelier [26]. These include: promoting active engagement; incrementally increasing task difficulty; providing verbal encouragement, motivation, feedback and praise; and offering variability in tasks. Below is the step-by-step procedure we use in our protocol and the corresponding principles of implementation. The video accompanying this paper illustrates the procedure in greater detail (http://pspb.org/client/Nursing.zip QuickTime Movie.)

1. Each participant has his/her own list of prescribed activities and an order in which they are to be implemented over the 30 minute session. This list is consulted every day for any possible changes. Activities are tailored to each participant's interests, abilities, and adjusted for problems with vision, hearing or language difficulties. The activities are organized in the order they will be given (easy to difficult). An activity cart can be used to organize and transport activities. Principle: treatment fidelity and variability in tasks.
2. The environment where the activities are to be implemented should be scanned to make sure it provides a good working space. Because attention is a problem in delirium, televisions, radios, pagers, and cell phones are turned off unless specifically a part of the session. The lighting level is adjusted so it is appropriate for the activities conducted; avoid areas where glare is a problem. Nursing and housekeeping staff are asked if they will need to provide care to participants or clean the space during the session. The idea is to reduce distracting interruptions and

ensure that the environment will support engagement in cognitive activities. Principle: control for extraneous factors that may affect the implementation of the intervention.

3. Upon entering the participant's room or the area where the session will take place, the interventionist should address the participant by his/her preferred name and sit down at his/her eye level. This approach reduces threat. The interventionist should be very cognizant of non-verbal communication: a pleasant manner is essential. The participant should be told the purpose of the session and their assent obtained: "Mrs. Jones, I am here to work with you on some games and activities. They may help in your rehabilitation. Would you like to do that now?" If the participant initially refuses, the interventionist should wait one hour and return to attempt assent. Principle: participant assent and proper communication technique.
4. Each participant should have time for needed bathroom visits prior to the intervention, assistive devices such as glasses/hearing aids should be worn, and complaints of pain should be addressed. Principle: ensure that the participant is maximally receptive to the cognitive activities.
5. Simple phrases, body language, gestures, and demonstration are used to communicate and promote understanding. The emotional expression of the participant, not simply his/her words, is important to note. The participant is not interrupted when speaking. Principle: proper communication technique.
6. The interventionists should speak slowly and never shout. Shouting makes it more difficult for older adults to hear what is being said because it raises the pitch of the voice. Principle: proper communication technique.
7. Implementation proceeds in this fashion: After introducing him- or herself and obtaining assent, the interventionist starts the timer and begins with the easiest level of task/exercise in the cognitive domain of attention. The level of difficulty is increased as success occurs with the simpler task. For example: in the domain of attention, if the participant successfully counts to 10 (easy level), the moderate level of difficulty is attempted by asking the participant to complete the Connect the Dots activity. If successful, the activity prescribed for the most difficult level in the domain of attention is then attempted. If at any point the participant is not able to complete a task/exercise, the interventionist should go on to the next cognitive domain and begin with an activity at the easy level, proceeding as described above. At least one task/exercise is attempted in each cognitive domain. The goal is to complete three activities (easy, moderate and difficult) in each cognitive domain. Principle: treatment fidelity, incremental increases in task difficulty and variability in tasks.
8. To initiate engagement in the activity the System of Least Restrictive Prompts is used [27]. The approach begins with verbal cueing: "Mrs. Jones, I'd like you to pick out all the items that are fruits in this picture." If there is no response, the interventionist uses both verbal cueing and demonstration of the activity: "Here is an apple. Now you try it." This system is only used to begin activities. If the participant continues to not respond, the approach in #10 is followed. Principle: active engagement and proper communication technique.
9. The interventionist works with each participant for 30 minutes or until he/she disengages from the activity. Disengagement is demonstrated by: dozing/falling

asleep, negative remarks about the activity, turning away from the interventionist/activity, asking to leave, leaving or attempting to leave the area. The interventionist may attempt to re-engage a participant three times by verbally prompting them to continue with the task/exercise. After the fourth disengagement the intervention is stopped. At the 30 minute point or after the fourth disengagement, the interventionist stops the timer and records the time. Principle: active engagement and treatment fidelity.

10. If the participant is too confused or refuses to initiate any activity, the intervention is not attempted at that time. Confusion can fluctuate throughout the day. The interventionist should return approximately one hour later to attempt a second session. If the participant is still too confused to participate in the activities, the activity is not attempted that day. Principle: active engagement and treatment fidelity.
11. During the activity, participants are given enough time to respond to the task/exercise. To aid communication, the same words are used when a question or a request is repeated; paraphrasing is avoided. Principle: proper communication technique.
12. Participants are encouraged to do as much as possible independently. Cueing is used as needed, however active involvement in the session is vital to improvement. The idea is to have the participant engage in cognitive activity that is sufficiently challenging to stimulate cognitive processing but not frustration. Principle: active engagement and treatment fidelity.
13. Praise is given freely. This feedback is very important because praise is a reward. Principle: feedback and praise.
14. Participants are encouraged/motivated throughout the session. For example: "You are doing well. Keep going!" Principle: verbal encouragement and motivation.
15. The activity should be fun and interesting. The interventionists should demonstrate enjoyment by his/her verbal and non-verbal communication. Principle: verbal encouragement and motivation
16. The interventionist ends the session by thanking the participant for his/her time and for an enjoyable afternoon. Principle: motivation and proper communication technique.
17. The time on task, level of participation and the activities attempted are recorded on the Engagement Rating Form. Principle: treatment fidelity
18. If for any reason the intervention was not implemented according to protocol, a Protocol Deviation Form is completed and the reason(s) for protocol deviation are indicated. Principle: treatment fidelity.

Conclusion

We are testing a novel non-pharmacological intervention for delirium in persons with dementia that, to our knowledge, has not been tested before in this population. Our intervention targets underlying cognitive problems, such as inattention, that are present in delirium regardless of cause. In this regard, the intervention has the potential to compliment other approaches to delirium resolution. We are encouraged by our pilot work on the development of this intervention [28] and are undertaking a larger project to improve care for people with dementia who suffer the devastating effects of delirium. We are sharing our practical protocol in the hope that it will be replicated and improved in other studies.

Competing Interests

The authors declare that they have no competing interests.

Authors' Contributions

All authors contributed to the development of the manuscript. AMK developed the intervention and the process for its implementation. LC assisted in the classification of activities by cognitive domain. NH and PM developed the script and were instrumental in the production of the video that accompanies this manuscript.

Acknowledgments

This study is supported by The National Institute of Nursing Research (NINR), the National Institutes of Health, grant number R01: NR012242. NINR had no role in study design; in the writing of the manuscript; or in the decision to submit the manuscript for publication.

Additional Information on Video

File name: Nursing

Format: http://pspb.org/client/Nursing.zip QuickTime Movie

Title of Data: Training session: Implementing Cognitively Stimulating Recreational Activities

Description of Data: Video illustration of implementing intervention

References

[1] American Psychiatric Association: *Diagnostic and Statistical Manual of Mental Disorders (DSM-IV)*. 4th edition. Washington, DC: American Psychiatric Press Inc.; 1994.

[2] Inouye SK: Delirium in older persons. *New England Journal of Medicine* 2006, 354(11):1157-1165.

[3] Fick DM, Agostini JV, Inouye SK: Delirium superimposed on dementia: A systematic review. *Journal of the American Geriatrics Society* 2002, 50(10):1723-1732.

[4] McCusker J, Cole M, Dendukuri N, Belzile E, Primeau F: Delirium in older medical inpatients and subsequent cognitive and functional status: A prospective study. *CMAJ: Canadian Medical Association Journal* 2001, 165(5):575-583.

[5] Ellul J, Archer N, Foy CM, Poppe M, Boothby H, Nicholas H, Brown RG, Lovestone S: The effects of commonly prescribed drugs in patients with Alzheimer's disease on the rate of deterioration. *Journal of Neurology, Neurosurgery and Psychiatry* 2007, 78(3):233-239.

[6] McShane R, Keene J, Gedling K, Fairburn C, Jacoby R, Hope T: Do neuroleptic drugs hasten cognitive decline in dementia? Prospective study with necropsy follow up. *British Medical Journal* 1997, 314(7076):266-270.

[7] Kolanowski A, Fick D, Clare L, Therrien B, Gill D: An intervention for delirium superimposed on dementia based on cognitive reserve theory. *Aging and Mental Health* 2010, 14(2): 232-242.

[8] Kolanowski, A, Fick, D, Litaker, M, Clare,L, Leslie, D, Boustani, M. Study protocol for the recreational stimulation for elders as a vehicle to resolve delirium superimposed on dementia. Trials [doi 10.1186/1745-6215-12-119], 12(119).

[9] Clare L, Woods RT. Cognitive training and cognitive rehabilitation for people with early-stage Alzheimer's disease: A review. *Neuropsychological Rehabilitation.* 2004;14:385-401.

[10] Richards M, Sacker A: Lifetime antecedents of cognitive reserve. *Journal of Clinical and Experimental Neuropsychology* 2003, 25(5):614-624.

[11] Savickas, M. The psychology of interests. In M. Savickas and A. Spokane (Eds) *Vocational interests*. Palo Alto: Davies-Black Publishing; 1999;19-56.

[12] Csikszentmihalyi, M., and Csikszentmihalyi, I. *Optimal experience: Psychological studies of flow in consciousness*. New York: Cambridge University Press; 1988.

[13] Choi J, Medalia A: Factors associated with a positive response to cognitive remediation in a community psychiatric sample. *Psychiatric Services* 2005, 56(5):602-604.

[14] Kolanowski AM, Litaker M, Buettner L: Efficacy of theory-based activities for behavioral symptoms of dementia. *Nursing Research* 2005, 54(4):219-228.

[15] Kolanowski A, Buettner L, Costa P: Capturing interests: Therapeutic recreation activities for persons with dementia. *Therapeutic Recreation Journal* 2001, 35(3): 220-236.

[16] Kolanowski A, Litaker M, Buettner, L, Moeller, J, Costa, P: A randomized clinical trial of theory-based activities for the behavioral symptoms of dementia in nursing home residents. *Journal of the American Geriatrics Society* in press.

[17] Blessed G, Tomlinson BE, Roth M. The association between quantitative measures of dementia and of senile change in the cerebral grey matter of elderly subjects. *British Journal of Psychiatry.* 1968;114(512):797-811.

[18] Hughes CP, Berg L, Danziger WL, Coben LA, Martin RL. A new clinical scale for the staging of dementia. *British Journal of Psychiatry.* 1982;140:566-572.

[19] Folstein MF, Folstein SE, McHugh PR. Mini-mental state: A practical method for grading the cognitive state of patients for the clinician. *Journal of Psychiatric Research.* 1975;12(3):189-198.

[20] Mahoney FI, Barthel DW. Functional evaluation: The Barthel Index. *Maryland State Medical Journal.* 1965;14:61-65.

[21] Buettner L, Martin SL. *Therapeutic recreation in the nursing home*. State College, PA: Venture Pub.; 1995.

[22] Riddick C, Keller M: Benefits of therapeutic recreation in gerontology. In *Benefits of therapeutic recreation: A consensus view*. Edited by Coyle C, Kinney W, Riley B, Shanks J. Philadelphia: Temple University, Therapeutic Recreation Program; 1991: 151-204.

[23] Buettner LL: Simple Pleasures: A multilevel sensorimotor intervention for nursing home residents with dementia. *American Journal of Alzheimer's Disease and Other Dementias* 1999, 14(1):41-52.

[24] Buettner L, Fitzsimmons S: Introduction to evidence-based recreational therapy. *Annual in Therapeutic Recreation* 2007, 15:12-90.

[25] Buettner L, Kolanowski A: Practice guidelines for recreation therapy in the care of people with dementia. *Geriatric Nursing* 2003, 24(1):18-23; quiz 24-15.

[26] Green CS, Bavelier D: Exercising your brain: A review of human brain plasticity and training-induced learning. *Psychology and Aging* 2008, 23(4):692-701.

[27] Engelman KK, Mathews RM, Altus DE: Restoring dressing independence in persons with Alzheimer's disease: A pilot study. *American Journal of Alzheimer's Disease and Other Dementias* 2002, 17(1):37-43.

Kolanowski AM, Fick DM, Clare L, Steis M, Boustani M, Litaker M: Pilot Study of a Nonpharmacological Intervention for Delirium Superimposed on Dementia. *Res. Gerontol. Nurs.*:1-7.

In: Non-Pharmacological Therapies ...
Editor: Elisabetta Farina
ISBN: 978-1-63321-860-4

Chapter 4

How Do People with Dementia and Their Carers Evaluate the Meeting Centers Support Programme?

***Rose-Marie Dröes*[1], *Franka J. M. Meiland*[1], *Mirjam J. Schmitz*[2] and *Willem van Tilburg*[3]**
[1] Department of Psychiatry and Department of Nursing Home Medicine, EMGO Institute for Health and Care Research, Alzheimer Center, VU University Medical Center, Amsterdam, Netherlands
[2] SEIN, Epilepsy Institute in the Netherlands, Heemstede, Netherlands
[3] Department of Psychiatry, EMGO Institute for Health and Care Research, VU University Medical Center, Amsterdam, Netherlands

Abstract

Background. The Meeting Centers Support Programme (MCSP) offers information and practical, emotional and social support to persons with dementia and their carers in local community centers. In this study the support programme was evaluated by participants (persons with dementia and carers) who utilized the MCSP for at least three months.

Methods. Data collection took place within the framework of an implementation study in 11 meeting centers. 148 persons with dementia and 148 carers participated in the study. Data were collected after three and seven months of participation by means of questionnaires.

Results. In general the persons with dementia and the carers were satisfied to very satisfied with the different elements of the support programme, the enrolment procedure, the contact with personnel, the location, and the facilities the centers have to offer. Half of the persons with dementia and one third of all carers indicated that they had made new acquaintances and friends at the center. Though satisfied with the programme, a majority of the persons with dementia (67% after three months and 58% after seven months) said that they were never asked what they wanted to do. The large majority of the carers feel somewhat less (42%) or much less (46%) burdened as a result of participating in the programme. This reduction of experienced burden proved to be related to satisfaction about the total programme ($r_s=0.35$, $p<0.005$), experienced understanding for the own situation in informative meetings (r_s=0.19, p= 0.05), and experienced emotional support in contacts with other carers (r_s=0.19, p=0.03).

Conclusion. The satisfaction of the persons with dementia and their carers about the MCSP, and the percentage of carers who experienced a reduction of burden thanks to the support they received are high. However, the fact that two thirds of the persons with dementia say that they were never asked what they want to do indicates that the methods used by the staff need to be improved.

Keywords: Dementia, carers, support programme, day care, respite, evaluation

Introduction

Over the past two decades many types of support have been developed for people with dementia and their family carers, ranging from respite care, discussion groups and informative meetings to various educational materials, such as books, information flyers, training courses and television documentaries. However, the development of the various types of support has also resulted in severe fragmentation of the offer (Hadderingh et al., 1991; Schulz, 1991; Van der Roest et al., 2008; Van Mierlo et al., 2010). As a consequence family carers, and even professional carers, sometimes can't see the wood for the trees, and therefore tend not to utilize the offered support. To counter these objections several care and welfare institutions in Amsterdam have, since 1993 and in cooperation with the department of Psychiatry of the VU University medical center (VUmc) in Amsterdam, combined their offer and expertise in the Meeting Centers Model (Dröes and Breebaart, 1994; Dröes, 1996; Dröes et al., 2000; 2004a,b).

This model represents a broad and integrated support programme for people with dementia and their carers, which is offered in low-threshold community centers and centers for the elderly by a small, permanent team of professionals (a programme coordinator, an activity therapist and a nursing assistant). The Meeting Centers Support Programme focuses on people with mild to moderate dementia who live in the community, and their carers. In addition to information, the programme aims to give them the practical, emotional and social support they need to cope with the consequences of dementia in their life. The support programme integrates several support activities for the person with dementia and his/her carer, that have been succesfully applied and evaluated in practice and/or research in the last decades (see also Dröes, 1997b; Dröes et al., 2004b; Finnema et al., 2000; Knight et al., 1993; Zarit et al., 1999; Pusey and Richards, 2001; Acton and Kang, 2001; Cooke et al., 2001; Smits et al., 2007; Van Mierlo et al., 2010).The persons with dementia are offered:

- A social club with special activity programmes, such as memory games, reading the newspaper, setting the table, listening to music, walking and making excursions, that can have a positive effect on cognitive functioning, e.g. recent memory (Karlsson et al., 1985; Spector et al., 2003), improved speech skills, initiative; alertness, and improved mood (e.g. Baker et al., 2001; Dröes, 1997a,b; Sandman et al., 1988);
- Psychosocial and emotion-oriented approaches, such as '*identifying pleasant activities'*, which has been shown to have a positive effect on mood (Teri et al., 1994); *emotion-oriented care*, e.g. Validation, which also can have a positive impact

on mood (Toseland et al., 1997; De Lange et al., 1999; Finnema et al., 2000); *reality orientation* and *cognitive stimulation*, which are associated with a slower cognitive decline (Mettitieri et al., 2001; Spector et al., 2003); *psychomotor therapy,* which has been shown to positively impact aggression, nighttime restlessness, general satisfaction (Dröes and Van Tilburg, 1996; Dröes, 1997a) and depressed mood (Teri et al., 2003); and *reminiscence,* which appears to positively influence cognitive functioning (Tadaka and Kanagawa, 2004), mood (Brooker and Duce, 2000; Gibson, 1994; Woods, 1996) and quality of life (Meguro et al., 2008), and
- Case management for the persons with dementia.

The carers are offered:

- Informative meetings, that help them to understand how to deal with the consequences of dementia (Brodaty et al., 1994);
- Discussion groups, to support the psychological and emotional adjustment and to prevent them from becoming overburdened (Brodaty and Gresham, 1998; Cuijpers, 1992; Morris et al., 1989);
- Respite care to prevent overburdening (Flint et al., 1995; Gaugler et al., 2003; Lawton et al., 1989), and
- A weekly consulting hour for practical and emotional support of individual carers (Mittelman et al., 1995, 1996; Vernooij-Dassen et al., 2000).

In addition, a monthly center meeting is organized during which all the people involved (persons with dementia, carers and professionals) can express their wishes concerning changes in the programme. The way in which the cooperating care and welfare institutions participate in carrying out the support programme has been laid down in a cooperation protocol.

The Meeting Centers model has spread to many other regions in the Netherlands and has shown to be implementable in all new locations (Dröes et al., 2004c; Meiland et al., 2004). The model has also been successfully applied in a meeting center for Surinamese elderly people with dementia and their family carers in Amsterdam (Osté and Dröes, 2004). At present a total of 70 meeting centers are operational in the Netherlands and another 20 are in preparation. In recent years meeting centers for persons with dementia and their carers have also been set up in other countries in and outside Europe, for example Aruba, Belgium, Italy and Surinam.

Research carried out by the VUmc over the periods 1994-1996 and 2000-2003 has shown that the combined support of the person with dementia and the family carer in meeting centers, as compared to regular day treatment, has a more positive effect on the behaviour and mood of people with dementia (less behaviour problems, especially less non-social behaviour and inactivity; less depressive behaviour, more self-esteem; tendency towards delayed nursing home admission) and the strength of the family carers (less experienced burden, keeping up the care for a longer period and at a better level); less psychological and psychosomatic symptoms in carers who feel lonely, more experienced support from professional institutions, expansion of social network (Dröes et al., 2000, 2004a, 2004b; 2006; Meiland et al., 2005). The average duration of participation before admission into a nursing home was 41.2 weeks in the meeting centers, as compared to 24.9 weeks in the regular day treatment group. This effect on delay of nursing home admission is repeated in the admission percentages. After seven months 4% of the people with dementia who participated in the Meeting Centers Support Programme had been admitted into a nursing home, whereas the percentage in the group that utilized regular day treatment was already 29% after seven months (Dröes et al., 2004a). The costs of the integrated support offered were no higher than the costs of the regular day treatment involved in this study. This means that for this group of clients (people with mild to moderately severe dementia and family carers who also want support) the meeting centers have considerably more effect for the same costs.

Evaluation of the support programme in the first Amsterdam Meeting Centers in 1996 showed that the majority of the people with dementia and their carers were satisfied about the support they received (Goffin et al., 1996). In this article we report on a large-scale evaluation of the Meeting Centers Support Programme among people with dementia and their carers who participated in the programme in eleven meeting centers in different regions of the Netherlands between 2000 and 2003. The study was carried out by the department of Psychiatry of the VU University medical center as part of an implementation study (Dröes et al., 2003).

Methods

Design

In order to assess the opinions of the people with dementia and their carers on the support they receive and on the various elements in the support programme, all new participants in the support programme who agreed to take part in the study were interviewed extensively on the different programme elements after three months and after seven months of participation.

Sample

The research took place in two older meeting centers in Amsterdam and in nine new meeting centers in other regions in the Netherlands (at that time all the meeting centers that existed in the Netherlands). All 172 people with dementia and their carers who over a period of eighteen months (Autumn 2000-Spring 2002) started participating in the support programme in these meeting centers, were invited to participate in the study by means of an informed consent procedure. 18 persons refused to participate in the study and 6 quit the programme within 3 weeks. Table 1 reflects the characteristics of the 148 people with dementia and their carers who in principle consented to participate in the study per region. A distinction has been made between 'follow-up' centers (operational for more than two years: the Amsterdam centers and Amstelveen) and 'starting' centers (operational for less than two years).

With regard to the people with dementia there were no significant differences between the regions on sex, age, civil status, severity of the dementia and physical disability. In all, about the same number of men and women came to the centers, the average age varied between 75 and 80, the majority were married or cohabited, had mild to moderately severe dementia and displayed a mild level of physical disability. Although the majority of the participants had Alzheimer's disease or suffered from another type of dementia, we observed some difference between the regions on other diagnoses, which was caused partly by variations in the admission policies of the individual meeting centers. In every center, according to the informal carers, at least half of the participants exhibited four or more psychiatric behaviour symptoms. Psychiatric symptoms most frequently present were apathy (73%), depression/dysphoria (67%), appetite and eating abnormalities (58%), and agitation/aggression (52%).

With regard to the family carers: in all regions the majority were women, married or cohabiting, and a minority were gainfully employed. Two-thirds cared for their spouses, 24% cared for their parents, and 10% had another relationship to the person with dementia. In general they shared a household with the person with dementia, or they lived in the same municipality. On average their age was between 60 and 70. An occasional exception showed a higher or lower average age. In nearly all centers the majority of family carers exhibited psychological and psychosomatic symptoms.

Of the 148 people with dementia and their carers who utilized the meeting centers at the start of the study, and from whom informed consent was received, 21 client dyads were excluded because they had been utilizing the meeting centers for longer than seven months (see figure 1). Of the remaining 127 dyads a first questionnaire was administered to 99 (78%) people with dementia and their carers, and a second questionnaire was administered to 104 (82%) people with dementia and 97 (76%) family carers. Both a first and a second questionnaire were administered to 92 (72%) people with dementia and 81 (64%) family carers.

Reasons for non-participation of people with dementia in the evaluation study were: they dropped out of the programme within three months (n=14), they had never actually participated in the programme (n=1), or the person was too severely aphasic to allow administering the questionnaire (n=1). Reasons for the carers not to participate in the study were: overburdened or ill (n=4), dropped out of the programme within three months (n=2), admitted into a nursing home, care facility or day treatment (n=4) and deceased (n=2).

Reasons for drop-out on the first questionnaires were: enrolled in the evaluation study too late, and questionnaire returned too late (11 people with dementia and 13 carers). One carer felt too overburdened to participate at the time of the first questionnaire. On one of the persons with dementia and two family carers there is no information why the first questionnaire was not administered (see figure 1). Reasons for drop-out on the second questionnaire were: refusal to participate further in the study, illness of the person with dementia or carer, transfer to day treatment or nursing home, and administering the second questionnaire too late.

In a number of cases (see figure 1) only the second questionnaire was filled out for the participants. There were two reasons: these people were not enrolled in the study until *after* the first three months, which made it impossible to administer the first questionnaire on time, or they returned the questionnaire long after the three months had passed.

Not all questions in the questionnaires were answered by all respondents. Some questions did not apply to some of them, because they had not made use of the evaluated elements of the support programme during the period in question.

Table 1. Characteristics of the people with dementia in starting Meeting centers (A-E) and the 'follow-up centers'(F,G) in the different regions

Region	*A(n=42)*	*B(n=18)*	*C(n=5)*	*D(n=9)*	*E(n=11)*	*Starters*		*F(n=14)*	*G(n=49)*	*Follow-up centers*	
Characteristic						χ^2	p			χ^2	p
Sex											
Male	23(54.8%)	8(44.4%)	3(60.0%)	5(55.6%)	4(36.4%)			9(64.3%)	33(67.3%)		
Female	19(45.2%)	10(55.6%)	2(40.0%)	4(44.4%)	7(63.6%)	1.72	0.79	5(35.7%)	16(32.7%)	0.05	0.83
Age (sd)	76.9(7.2)	77.5(6.8)	79.0(4.1)	75.1(6.4)	79.5(5.8)	F=0.66	0.62	75.1(3.0)	75.6(9.6)	t=-0.20	0.84
Civil status											
Married/cohabiting	28(66.7%)	11(61.1%)	2(40.0%)	8(88.9%)	5(45.5%)			11(78.6%)	37(75.5%)		
Divorced/widow(er)	14(33.3%)	7(38.9%)	3(60.0%)	1(11.1%)	6(54.5%)	5.47	0.24	3(21.4%)	12(24.5%)	0.06	0.81
Diagnosis											
Dementia											
Alzheimer type	23(54.8%)	10(55.6%)	2(40.0%)	7(77.8%)	6(54.5%)			5(35.7%)	25(51.0%)		
Vascular	4(9.5%)	1(5.6%)	1(20.0%)	-	2(18.2%)			1(7.1%)	4(8.2%)		
Mixed type	3(7.1%)	1(5.6%)	-	1(11.1%)	-			4(28.6%)	8(16.3%)		
Other type	8(19.0%)	1(5.6%)	-	-	2(18.2%)	18.90	0.02*	2(14.3%)	6(12.2%)	3.76	0.15
Amnestic syndrome											
Memory disorders	-	4(22.2%)	-	-	1(9.1%)			1(7.1%)	-		
Other											
Depression	1(2.4%)	-	-	1(11.1%)	-			-	1(2.0%)		
Unknown	3(7.1%)	1(5.6%)	2(40.0%)	-	-			1(7.1%)	5(10.2%)		
Severity of dementia											
Forgetfulness	1(2.4%)	2(11.1%)	-	-	-			1(7.1%)	-		
Early stage dementia	9(21.4%)	1(5.6%)	-	2(22.2%)	2(18.2%)			2(14.3%)	4(8.2%)		
Mild dementia	11(26.2%)	5(27.8%)	2(40.0%)	1(11.1%)	6(54.5%)			3(21.4%)	5(10.2%)		
Moderate dementia	10(23.8%)	7(38.9%)	2(40.0%)	2(22.2%)	1(9.1%)	17.24	0.64	5(35.7%)	17(34.7%)	6.38	0.27
Mod. severe dementia	9(21.4%)	3(16.7%)	1(20.0%)	3(33.3%)	2(18.2%)			3(21.4%)	10(20.4%)		
Severe dementia	2(4.8%)	-	-	1(11.1%)	-			-	7(14.3%)		
Unknown	-	-	-	-	-			-	6(12.2%)		
NPI											
total score (sd)	26.1(15.2)	25.8(14.0)	-	23.6(20.5)	28.3(15.9)	F=0.46	0.71	11.0(6.13)	26.9(16.28)	t=-3.54	0.01*
NPI-score ≥4											
behaviour symptoms	30(71.4%)	14(77.8%)	-	7(77.8%)	7(63.6%)	1.25	0.74	7(50.0%)	27(55.1%)	2.41	0.12

*p≤ 0.05. A=Amstelland & De Meerlanden; B=Groningen; C=Haarlem; D=Nieuwegein; E=Nijmegen; F=Amstelveen; G=Amsterdam De Pijp & Buitenveldert; NPI=Neuropsychiatric Inventory.

Persons with dementia n=148	Clients in Meeting Centers that consented to participate in the study	Carers n=148
n=37	Excluded or drop-out within 3 months	n=33
n=21	more than 7 months utilization of Meeting center at the start of the study	n=21
n=16	other reasons (see text)	n=12
n=99	Questionnaire 1	n=99
	Reasons for drop-out	
n=11	enrolled too late for questionnaire 1 or returned questionnaire too late	n=13
--	overburdened	n=1
n=1	unknown	n=2
n=104	Questionnaire 2	n=97
n=12	only questionnaire 2 completed	n=16
n=92	both questionnaires completed	n=81
	Reasons for drop-out	
n=2	refusal/not returned	n=6
n=2	illness of person with dementia	n=3
--	illness of carer	n=4
n=1	transferred to day treatment	n=3
n=1	transferred to nursing home	n=2
n=1	questionnaire administered too late	n=2

Figure 1. Numbers of persons with dementia and their carers who participated in the evaluation study, and reasons for drop out during the study.

Measuring Instruments and Procedure

After the person with dementia and the carer had agreed to take part in the study at the start of their participation in the support programme, trained interviewers gathered background characteristics of the person with dementia and the carer in an interview with the carer, based on a standardized list of questions (see table 1). To determine the severity of the dementia the Dutch version of Reisberg's Global Deterioration Scale (Reisberg, 1983; Muskens, 1993) was used (α=0.90). The scale was filled out by the general practitioner or the programme coordinator of the meeting centers one month after the person with dementia joined the programme, and after discussing his/her home functioning with his carer. To inventory behaviour problems and psychological problems in the person with dementia we used the NeuroPsychiatric Inventory (NPI; Cummings et al., 1994; Kat et al., 2002; α=0.88). With regard to the variables 'feeling of competence', and 'somatic complaints' of the carer we used the modified version of the Feeling of Competence Scale (Teunisse and De Haan, 1994; α=0.79) and the subscale Somatic complaints of the General Health Questionnaire (GHQ-28, Goldberg and Hillier 1978). The latter three lists were completed by the carer by means of interviews.

In connection with the programme evaluation all new participants in the support programme received an evaluation questionnaire after three months and after seven months of participation, over a period of eighteen months. The questionnaire for the *people with dementia* consisted of 13 questions and focused on, among other things, the following topics: location, staff, atmosphere, food and beverages, the activities, opportunities to take the initiative in the center, social contacts gained at the center and influence on the programme and its execution. The evaluation questionnaire for the *carers* consisted of 30 questions related to, among other things: reason for participation in the support programme, satisfaction regarding the enrolment procedure and intake procedure, opinion on the informative meetings, discussion groups, consulting hour, social club and monthly center meeting, satisfaction regarding the entire support programme, feelings of burden, experienced emotional and practical support from other participating carers, contacts gained at the meeting center, participation in public activities at the community center.

The people with dementia were interviewed at the meeting center, and the carers received their questionnaires through the mail. In the earlier Amsterdam Study we already gained experience with administering these questionnaires (Dröes, 1996). During that study it proved quite possible for the persons with dementia to answer the questions. For some questions we used text cards to help people to concentrate on the subject being discussed.

The carers were asked to complete the questionnaire anonymously and without interference from the staff members at the meeting centers, and to return them directly to the researchers. This procedure was chosen to avoid carers giving socially desirable answers. The questionnaires were coded, in order to be able to determine the relationship between background characteristics and answers in the questionnaires in analyses. The codes were known only to the researcher and the project leader.

Analysis

For the data analysis we used the SPSS-Windows 10.1 programme.

The gathered background characteristics were represented by means of descriptive statistics and compared between the centers with Chi^2 and t-tests (see Table 1).

To determine whether the eleven meeting centers could be treated as one homogeneous group in the analysis, we used the Kruskal Wallis test and tested whether they differed significantly on the variables 'severity of the dementia', 'the feeling of competence', and 'somatic symptoms of the carer'. All tests were conducted with a 5% significance level. We investigated what the reasons for drop-out had been during the research period.

Finally, we calculated the percentages for the results of the evaluation questionnaires, and Spearman rank correlations were calculated to determine the correlation between the satisfaction of carers about the support programme and the experienced burden and support.

Results

The Kruskal Wallis test showed that there were no significant differences between the meeting centers on severity of the dementia or on feeling of competence and somatic complaints of the carers. We therefore treated them as one homogeneous group in the further analysis.

Satisfaction of the Persons with Dementia

The persons with dementia were very positive about the day/social club in both the first and the second questionnaire (see table 2).

Table 2. Satisfaction of the persons with dementia with the social club after three (questionnaire 1) and after seven months (questionnaire 2) of participation. The data are presented in absolute figures and percentages (n_1=99, n_2=104)

Content	Questionnaire 1			Questionnaire 2		
	very satisfied	satisfied	not satisfied	very satisfied	satisfied	not satisfied
Social club	33(34%)	59(62%)	4 (4%)	38(39%)	58(59%)	2(2%)
Activities	21(23%)	70(77%)	0 (0%)	26(28%)	67(71%)	1(1%)

In the first questionnaire only a few of them indicated being dissatisfied with the atmosphere (n=2), the quality of the facilities (n=3) and the quality of the food (n=2). Ten participants were not satisfied with the size of the space of the social club and the number of staff, 90% expressed satisfaction on these points. All participants were satisfied with the contact with the staff, and 96% felt the staff really listened to them. The results of the second questionnaire showed comparable results.

In both questionnaires 95% of the participants indicated they felt they could do what they enjoyed in the social club. The same is shown in their satisfaction regarding the *offer of activities*. Activities they enjoyed or even enjoyed very much (after three and seven months of participation respectively) were: psychomotor therapy (82%, 81%), listening to music (80%, 85%), and playing games (80%, 83%). Activities such as reading the newspaper (78%, 80%), setting the table and washing the dishes (60%, 59%), memory games (67%, 73%) and excursions (71%, 85%) were also judged positively by many of the participants. Least enjoyed were: drawing (35%, 50%) and shopping (42%, 34%), although a relatively large group still enjoyed these activities. The participants responded to the question which activity they liked most with a wide variety of answers. The most frequently mentioned activities were: walking (22%) and listening to music (20%).

Of the participants 67% in the first questionnaire and 58% in the second questionnaire said that they were never asked what they wanted, 23% (and 25%) said they were sometimes asked and the rest said they were often or always asked (10%, 17%). Only one of the participants who said they were asked what they want indicated at the first evaluation that the staff subsequently did not do what he wanted (at the second evaluation nobody said this). The others (26%, 32%) said that the group would sometimes or frequently/always (71%, 68%) do what they wanted. In answer to the question whether they would like to do or learn something they had not done so far in the social club, 22 participants responded affirmatively at the first evaluation, as did 20 participants at the second evaluation. They mentioned various games (pool, play cards, chess, bridge, memory games), outdoor activities (football, walking, visiting museums, bicycle ride), creative activities (do fretwork, painting, fancywork, handicrafts, singing) and computer games or being able to use a library. All of these suggestions were passed on to the staff and several of the mentioned activities were integrated in the programme.

When asked about participation in the monthly center meetings, 22% indicated this was important; at the time of the second evaluation this percentage had increased to 31%. Many of the participants indicated they did not participate in the center meetings (29%, 34%), or they did not know whether they attended these meetings or not (34%, 20%). The other participants felt it was not important or it did not apply to them. Only one participant indicated that people did not listen to his opinion during the meeting, the others indicated they did not know (60%) or they felt that people listened sufficiently or very well (38%). The results of the second evaluation pointed in the same direction.

Half of the participants indicated in the first and the second questionnaire that they had made new acquaintances and friends at the social club. 31 participants (31%), and 32 participants (31%) actually described one or more persons in the first and second questionnaire respectively.

There was room for comments at the end of the questionnaires. We present a few here: ‘fantastic people, relaxed atmosphere, wonderful we can participate’. ‘no complaints, I enjoy it’, ‘at first I didn’t feel like going, but now I really enjoy it’, ‘admiration for the people who work here’, ‘when you come here every week, you enjoy it; I always make jokes’, ‘most games are too slow due to the slow pace of the other participants’, ‘I enjoy going to the meeting center’, ‘don’t change too much at the club, it is fine the way it is!’.

The overall satisfaction with the social club and the activities was not related to the severity of dementia (social club first evaluation r_s=0.11, p=0.30; second evaluation rs=0.02, p= 0.88; activities first evaluation r_s=0.09, p=0.42; second evaluation rs=0.12, p= 0.27) nor to the number of neuropsychiatric symptoms (social club first evaluation r_s=0.12, p=0.32; second evaluation r_s=0.09, p= 0.41; activities first evaluation r_s=-0.08, p=0.52; second evaluation rs=-0.08, p= 0.50) at baseline.

Satisfaction of the Carers

The Enrolment Procedure

The questions on the enrolment procedure were completed by 108 family carers (97 at the first evaluation, and 11 of those who only filled out the second evaluation questionnaire). Apart from three respondents who were moderately satisfied, all carers were satisfied to very satisfied with the procedure (accessibility of programme coordinator, information on the support programme and introduction in the meeting center). Although most carers were satisfied with the waiting time and cooperation of the GP, 13% said they had experienced the waiting time as (too) long, and 25% judged the cooperation of the GP as moderate to poor.

Informative Meetings

Of the 79 carers who attended the informative meetings only two expressed being moderately satisfied, the others were *satisfied* or very satisfied (see Table 3). In the second questionnaire one participant was dissatisfied and five participants were moderately satisfied.

Most carers (79%) judged the offered *quantity of information* during these meetings as sufficient or good, 5% felt it was too little, and 3% said it was too much. The second questionnaire also showed general satisfaction with the quantity of information, 7% felt that not enough information was offered.

Most carers (97%, 99%) also expressed in both questionnaires that there was sufficient *opportunity to ask questions.*

Table 3. Satisfaction of carers about the informative meetings, discussion group and the support programme as a whole at the time of the first and second questionnaires. The data are presented in absolute numbers and in percentages

Content	*Questionnaire 1*			*Questionnaire 2*		
	(very) satisfied	moderately satisfied	not satisfied	(very) satisfied	moderately satisfied	not satisfied
Informative meetings	77(97%)	2(3%)	0(0%)	73(92%)	5(7%)	1(1%)
Discussion group	71(92%)	5(7%)	1(1%)	70(91%)	4(5%)	3(4%)
Total Programme	93(98%)	2(2%)	0(0%)	90(95%)	5(5%)	0(0%)

Table 4. Carer judgement on the frequency of the various elements of the support programme at the first and the second measurements (questionnaires). The number of respondents is presented in absolutes and percentages

Frequency	*Questionnaire 1*			*Questionnaire 2*		
	too high	sufficient	too low	too high	sufficient	too low
Informative meetings	21(27%)	57(73%)	0(0%)	26(34%)	50(66%)	0(0%)
Discussion group	25(33%)	51(67%)	0(0%)	23(31%)	51(68%)	1(1%)
Consulting hour	23(29%)	56(70%)	1(1%)	24(28%)	57(67%)	4(5%)
Monthlymeeting	15(17%)	73(82%)	1(1%)	18(21%)	68(78%)	1(1%)

Many carers felt the information offered was *practicable:* in the first and second questionnaire 93% and 95% respectively indicated they used the offered information at home. In addition almost all respondents (except two in the first, and one in the second questionnaire) said they experienced more or less *understanding of their own situation.*

Regarding the *frequency* of the informative meetings: about one third found it was too high in both evaluations, the others were satisfied with the frequency (see Table 4). The meetings that addressed: 'Introduction to the dementia syndrome', 'Information on support services', 'Types of dementia', and 'Coping with behaviour problems' received the highest rating with regard to content.

The Discussion Group

Of the 79 carers 77 gave an opinion on the discussion group in the first questionnaire and 79 in the second. The large majority, in both evaluations, said they were (very) *satisfied* (see Table 3). To the question whether they received *emotional support* from the other carers in the discussion group, 31% said during the first evaluation they had experienced much support, 63% said they had received sufficient support, 7% said they had received insufficient or no support. In the second evaluation 31% said they had received much support, and 56% judged it as sufficient. During both evaluations nearly all (99% and 94%) carers indicated that they had received sufficient or much support from the person who chaired these meetings, and most carers felt they got practical advice (89% and 85% respectively). A vast majority (99% and 95%) indicated in both evaluations that the chairmanship was sufficient to good.

In both evaluations a majority (see Table 4) also expressed satisfaction regarding the *frequency* of the discussion group meetings (which varied in the different regions and was once every two, three or four weeks).

In the first evaluation 86% said the *size* of the group was satisfactory, in the second evaluation this had increased to 87%. In both evaluations five carers felt the group was too large.

The Consulting Hour

Of the 26 carers in the first evaluation and the 17 carers in the second evaluation who said they used the consulting hour on their own initiative, 17 and 13 respectively had contacted the programme coordinator by telephone regularly to frequently. Six and nine of them respectively came to the consulting hour at the meeting center regularly to frequently. Reasons the carers gave for utilizing the consulting hour were, in order of frequency: practical advice (57% in both questionnaires), discussing personal problems (54% and 60.7% respectively) and general information (46% and 46% respectively). In several cases the programme coordinator invited the carer to discuss the care of the person with dementia (34% and 39% respectively), or to discuss personal problems of the carer (29% and 39% respectively).

The Social Club

During the first evaluation 92% of the carers judged the *opening hours* of the social club as sufficient to good. At the time of the second evaluation this percentage decreased to 84%.

Most of the carers (80% and 74% respectively) indicated in both evaluations that they felt the *activities* for the participants in the social club were activating in a positive sense. The others responded to this question with 'I don't know'.

Approximately half of the carers indicated the *furnishing* of the space was inviting (58% and 54% respectively), others said the space was functional (33% and 37% respectively) and a small group felt the space was uninviting (5% and 5%). In both evaluations the majority

(87% and 84%) expressed satisfaction with the *size of the space*. Those who were not satisfied generally felt the space was too small. A very large part of the carers (93% and 93% in the first and second evaluation respectively) rated the *facilities* in the social club as sufficient to good. In both evaluations a large part of the carers (75% and 86%) were satisfied with the *transportation* to the social club.

In the first evaluation nearly everybody rated the social club's *contactability by phone*, the *number* and *the professionalism* of the staff as sufficient to good (99%, 98%, and 98% respectively). This was also the case in the second evaluation. Satisfaction on the degree of professionalism of the staff had even increased to 100% at that time. In the first evaluation almost all of the carers (93%) rated *communication with the staff* as good or sufficient (8%). In the second questionnaire satisfaction on this point had decreased somewhat: 86% still rated communication as good, and 14% said it was sufficient. In both evaluations a large majority (92%) felt they received sufficient *information* on the functioning of the person with dementia at the social club.

The Monthly Center Meeting

Three months after the start of participation in the support programme, a large part of the carers (76%) had participated at least one time in the monthly center meeting, and felt this meeting enhanced the involvement in the meeting center (86%) They furthermore felt that it offers the opportunity to discuss all kinds of matters (82%). After seven months of participation these percentages had barely changed. Only the number of carers who felt that the meetings enhanced involvement in the meeting center had increased (92%). A large majority of the carers (82% and 76% respectively) rated the frequency of the monthly meetings as good, a minority felt it was too high.

In both evaluations a large part of the carers (81% and 85% respectively) said the monthly center meeting made them feel they shared responsibility for the person with dementia with others.

Satisfaction with the Support, Experienced Burden and Emotional Support

Satisfaction

In the first evaluation 52% said they were satisfied with the total support programme, and 46% were very satisfied (see Table 3). Only 2% were moderately satisfied with the offered support. The percentages were almost identical in the second evaluation (48% and 46% respectively). The percentage of carers who were moderately satisfied had increased slightly at the second evaluation.

Burden

After three months most carers said they already felt less burdened than before they participated in the support programme (57% somewhat less, and 36% much less). After seven months the percentage that said they felt *much* less burdened had increased to 46%, while 42% said they felt somewhat less burdened.

Emotional support

Between three months and seven months of participation an increasing number of carers (41% and 89%) indicated experiencing *emotional support* in their contacts with other carers.

Relationship between Satisfaction with Programme, Experienced Burden and Emotional Support

The calculation of Spearman rank correlations showed that there was a statistically significant correlation between the reduction of experienced burden on the one hand, and satisfaction about the total support programme (first evaluation r_s=0.18, p=0.04; second evaluation r_s=0.35, p<0.005), experienced understanding for own situation in informative meetings (first evaluation r_s=0.23, p=0.03; second evaluation r_s=0.19, p= 0.05), and experienced emotional support in contacts with other carers (second evaluation r_s=0.19, p=0.03) on the other hand.

Relationship between Satisfaction with Programme and Baseline Data on Severity of Dementia and Neuropsychiatric Symptoms

Spearman rank correlations showed that there was no relation between overall satisfaction with the programme and severity of dementia at baseline (first evaluation r_s=0.08, p=0.52; second evaluation r_s=0.16, p= 0.12), or with the total number of neuropsychiatric symptoms at baseline (first evaluation r_s=-0.12, p=0.33; second evaluation r_s=-0.01, p= 0.95).

Expansion of Social Contacts of Carers

Finally, the questionnaires contained questions about the contacts between carers in and outside the meetings center, and other contacts they had gained at the community center. In the first evaluation 18% said that they had had contact by telephone with other carers once, various times or regularly. The total percentage in the second evaluation had increased to 27%.

A few carers (10%) said during the first evaluation that they had visited another carer. In the second evaluation this number had also increased to 17%. In the first evaluation only 2% of the carers had met another carer outside their homes. In the second evaluation this percentage had increased to 8%. In both evaluations only a very small percentage (6% and 2% respectively) had undertaken an activity with another carer once or various times.

On a group level, a substantial part of the carers in both evaluations indicated they experienced their contacts with other carers in the meeting center as an expansion of their circle of acquaintances (32% and 35% respectively). After three months seven carers had gained new contacts with other people at the community center (outside the support programme), after seven months their number had increased to eight. 25% of these carers said in the first evaluation that they appreciated these contacts as an expansion of their circle of acquaintances, in the second evaluation this percentage had grown to 63%.

Conclusion

This evaluation study among the participants with dementia and their carers shows that in general they are satisfied to very satisfied with the support they have received, the enrolment procedure, the location where the meeting center is organized, and the facilities the centers have to offer.

A large majority of the persons with dementia enjoy the activities offered in the social club, and half of them experience the contacts at the meeting center as an expansion of their circle of acquaintances. The least enjoyed activities, though still enjoyed by one third to one half of the participants, were drawing and shopping. This may be caused by personal preferences, but also by beginning apractic symptoms and disorientation problems. We saw comparable preferences for particular activities, such as walking and listening to music, in the first Amsterdam Meeting Centers study (Goffin et al., 1996). The fact that two thirds of the participants in the social club said that they were never asked what they want is remarkable. This requires a modification of the methods used by the staff, regardless of whether this result is an accurate reflection of reality. The participants clearly experience it this way. Acton c.s. (1999), Woods (2001), Dröes et al. (2006) and Gerritsen et al. (2010), among others, recommend (professional) carers of persons with dementia to pay more explicit attention to the communication with the person with dementia and to his/her personal perspective. This recommendation may also be valuable for meeting center staff, despite the fact that they already utilize various emotion- and experience-oriented approaches. A large majority of carers assessed the communication with the personnel as good, although satisfaction decreased somewhat between three and seven months of participation. This may have been caused by the fact that after seven months of participating in the programme carers have had more opportunities to get in contact with the personnel and had more experiences with them than after three months, resulting in more varied opinions on the commmunication.

In general the carers judge the *informative meetings* as positive, feel that the information offered is practicable, and experience understanding for their own situation during the meetings. However, one third of the carers feel the frequency of once every two weeks is too high. This may be caused by the fact that they feel quite burdened and therefore experience their time as precious when the person with dementia is in the meeting center. Some people actually express they prefer to take a break or do something for themselves.

All carers experienced support in the *discussion groups*, especially from the chairperson, but for a large part also from other carers. This is also something we observed before in the Amsterdam Meeting Centers (Goffin et al., 1996). As was the case regarding the informative meetings, approximately one third of the participants felt the frequency of the discussion group meetings is too high.

By no means did all carers utilize the weekly (telephonic) *consulting hour*. The majority did not feel the need to do so or discussed their problems with the programme coordinator at some other time. Those who did (approximately one third) generally had regular to frequent contact with the programme coordinator. The most important reasons for the contact were: personal problems of the carer, practical advice on caring for the person with dementia and general information.

A vast majority of the carers is positive about the *social club* with regard to the offered activities, size of the space, transportation to the club, the facilities, and communication with, number and professionalism of the meeting center staff. Opinion are divided on the furnishing: approximately half of the carers felt the furnishing is inviting, one third characterize it as functional, and a few people said it was uninviting. An important subject that deserves special attention in the future, in our opinion, because of the influence that the design of the environment can have on the functioning and mood of people with dementia (see also Day et al., 2000). Compared to the carers of the first Amsterdam Meeting Centers, the carers in the current centers felt more frequently that the offer is activating for the participants with dementia (74-80% now compared to 50-60% then) (Goffin et al., 1996).

A large part of the carers regularly participated in the monthly *center meeting* and said this makes them feel they are sharing responsibility for the person with dementia with others.

Satisfaction of the carers with the support programme as a whole (98% are satisfied to very satisfied) is extremely high. The percentages regarding the reduced experience of burden (93% first evaluation, 88% second evaluation) are also high. The correlation between less experienced burden on the one hand and satisfaction with the total support programme, the experienced understanding for the own situation during the informative meetings, and experiencing emotional support in contacts with other carers on the other hand, was also observed in the study of the first Amsterdam Meeting Centers (Goffin et al., 1996). However, the relationship found there between the reduction of experienced burden, utilization of the consulting hour and experiencing the contacts at the meeting centers as an expansion of the circle of acquaintances, are not confirmed in this current multi-center study.

As in the first Amsterdam Meeting Centers, contacts between carers gradually increase in the new centers, and approximately one third of all carers experienced the contacts in the meeting center as an expansion of their personal circle of acquaintances. Around 10% of them visited each other at home or had telephone contact, but they rarely undertook other activities together. The reason for this, besides a lack of spare time due to the burdensome care task, could be that most (younger) carers have their own friends to undertake activities with.

All in all we may conclude that the satisfaction of the persons with dementia and their carers about the support they received at the meeting centers is high. When there is some dissatisfaction, as for example about the frequency of several programme elements and the furnishing of the space, it is only in a minority of the participants. The results of this multi-center study furthermore confirm the results of earlier research conducted in the first Meeting Centers in Amsterdam.

In satisfaction surveys there is a real risk that the respondents will give socially desirable answers (Lewis, 1994; Forbes and Neufeld, 1997; Edwards et al., 2004). We have tried to prevent this by administering the questionnaire to the carers in writing, anonymously and without interference of the meeting center staff, and by asking a wide variety of questions at two measurement points (after three and seven months) and qualifying the possible answers when possible. We also chose to interview not only the carers, but also the persons with dementia, as increasingly recommended in the literature (Zarit et al., 1999; Woods, 2001; Clare, 2002a,b; Dröes, 2007; Gerritsen et al., 2010). Many of them proved willing to participate in the study. In our opinion, both of their judgements about the support programme, from each of their respective perspectives, together provide a sound and differentiated picture of the satisfaction of the users of the meeting centers about the support and assistance they received. Finally, we also compared the results of our study with those of the first Amsterdam Meeting Centers in 1996 and found that most of the results confirmed the earlier findings.

The results of this evaluation study are innovative as studies in which people with dementia are directly involved in the evaluation of a support programme in which they participated are still scarce (Smits et al., 2007; Van Mierlo et al., 2010). People were not excluded in advance based on the severity of their dementia. Most people were indeed able to give their opinion on the different questions, especially those posed in the present tense (e.g. how do you like the room, the personnel, the atmosphere, what activities at the club do you like?). Occasionally people had difficulty understanding a question. This was especially the case with the question on the monthly center meeting, in which activities conducted at the club are discussed by the personnel, the people with dementia and the carers. Some of the people with dementia did not remember they had participated in these meetings.

The positive results of this evaluation among people with dementia and their carers, in combination with the evidence on the surplus value of the meeting centers as compared to regular day care in nursing homes, i.e. improved behaviour, mood, and delay of admission into a nursing home of the persons with dementia and increase of feelings of competence of the carers described earlier (Dröes et al., 2000, 2004a, 2004b), not only confirm that combined interventions for people with dementia and their carer generally are more effective than single interventions (Acton and Kang, 2001; Dröes et al., 2004; Smits et al., 2007), but also show that they can be experienced as highly satisfactory by all parties. These results are more than sufficient reason to recommend the further dissemination of the Meeting Centers Support Programme, especially since combined, long-term and comprehensive interventions for people with dementia and their carers are still not common practice in many countries. The results of this evaluation study can help care and welfare organizations to set up and implement new meeting centers for people with dementia and their carers which are genuinely based on their needs and wishes.

References

Acton GJ and Kang J. (2001). Interventions to reduce the burden of caregiving for an adult with dementia: a meta-analysis. *Research in Nursing and Health*, 24(5): 349-360.

Acton GJ, Mayhew PA, Hopkins BA, Yauk S. (1999). Communicating with individuals with dementia. The impaired person's perspective. *J. Gerontol. Nurs.*, 25(2): 6-13.

Baker, R., Bell, S., Baker, E., Gibson, S., Holloway, J., Pearce, R., Dowling, Z., Thomas, P., Assey, J., Wareing, L.A., (2001). A randomized controlled trial of the effects of multi-sensory stimulation (MSS) for people with dementia. *Br. J. Clin. Psychol.*, 40, 81–96.

Brodaty H, Gresham M. (1989). Effect of a training programme to reduce stress in carers of patients with dementia. *BMJ,* 299: 1375-1379.

Brodaty H, Roberts K, Peters K. (1994). Quasi-experimental evaluation of an educational model for dementia caregivers. *Int. J. Geriatr. Psychiatry*, 9: 195-204.

Brooker, D.J.R., Duce, L., 2000. Well-being and activity in dementia: a comparison of group reminiscence therapy, structured goal-directed group activity and unstructured time. *Aging Ment. Health,* 4, 354–358.

Clare, L. (2002a). Developing awareness about awareness in early-stage dementia: The role of psychosocial factors. Dementia: *The International Journal of Social Research and Practice*, 1, 295-312.

Clare, L. (2002b). We'll fight it as long as we can: coping with the onset of Alzheimer's disease. *Aging and Mental Health*, 6, 139-148.

Cooke DD, McNally L, Mulligan KT, Harrison MJG, Newman SP. (2001). Psychosocial interventions for caregivers of people with dementia: a systematic review. *Aging Ment Health,* 5(2): 120-135.

Cummings JL, Mega M, Gray K, Rosenberg-Thompson S, Carusi DA, Gornbein J. (1994). The Neuropsychiatric Inventory: comprehensive assessment of psychopathology in dementia. *Neurology*, 44: 2308-2314.

Cuijpers P. (1992). De effecten van ondersteuningsgroepen voor verzorg(st)ers van dementerende ouderen thuis: een literatuuroverzicht. *Tijdschrift voor Gerontologie en Geriatrie*, 23: 12-17.

Day K, Carreon D, Stump C. (2000). The therapeutic design of environments for people with dementia: a review of the empirical research. *Gerontologist,* 40(4): 397-416.

Dröes RM. (1991). In Beweging; over psychosociale hulpverlening aan demente ouderen. [In Movement; on psychosocial care for the demented elderly.] Intro: Nijkerk.

Dröes RM. (ed). (1996). Amsterdamse Ontmoetingscentra; een nieuwe vorm van ondersteuning voor mensen met dementie en hun verzorgers.Thesis Publishers: Amsterdam.

Dröes RM. (1997a).. Psychomotor group therapy for demented patients in the nursing home. In: *Care-Giving in Dementia: Research and Applications*. Volume 2, Miesen BML, Jones GMM (eds.). Routledge: London/New York; 95-118.

Dröes RM. (1997b). Psychosocial treatment for demented patients; methods and effects. In: *Care-giving in dementia*. Vol. 2. (eds. B. Miesen and G. Jones) Routledge: UK.

Dröes, R.M. (2007). Insight in coping with dementia; listening to the voice of those who suffer from it. *Aging and Mental Health*, 11(2):115-118.

Dröes, R.M., Boelens-Van der Knoop, E.C.C., Bos, J., Meihuizen, L., Ettema, T.P., Gerritsen, D.L., Hoogeveen, F., Lange, J. de, Schölzel-Dorenbos, C. (2006). Quality of life in dementia in perspective; an explorative study of variations in opinions among people with dementia and their professional caregivers, and in literature. *Dementia: The International Journal of Social Research and Practice*, 5(4): 533-558.

Dröes RM, Breebaart E. (1994). Amsterdamse Ontmoetingscentra; een nieuwe vorm van ondersteuning voor dementerende ouderen en hun verzorgers. Voorstudie. Thesis Publishers: Amsterdam.

Dröes RM, Breebaart E, Meiland FJM, Tilburg W van, Mellenbergh GJ. (2004a). Effect of Meeting Centers Support Programme on feeling of competence of family caregivers and delay of institutionalization of people with dementia. *Aging Ment Health*, 8(3): 201-211.

Dröes RM, Breebaart E, Tilburg W van, Mellenbergh GJ. (2000). The effect of integrated family support versus day care only on behavior and mood of patients with dementia. *Int. Psychogeriatr,* 12(1): 99-116.

Dröes RM, Goffin JJM, Breebaart E, Rooij E de, Vissers H, Bleeker JAC, Tilburg W van. (2004d). Support programmes for caregivers of people with dementia: A review of methods and effects. In: Miesen B, Jones G. (eds.) *Caregiving in Dementia*, 3: 214-239.

Dröes RM, Meiland FJM, Schmitz MJ, Boerema I, Derksen E, Lange J de, Vernooij-Dassen MJFJ, Tilburg W van. (2004c). Variations in meeting centers for people with dementia and their carers: results of a multi-center implementation study. *Arch. Gerontol. Geriatr*, suppl. 9: 127-148.

Dröes RM, Meiland FJM, Schmitz M, Tilburg W van. (2004b). Effect of combined support for people with dementia and carers versus regular day care on behaviour and mood of persons with dementia: results from a multi-center implementation study. *Int. J. GeriatrPsychiatry*, 19: 1-12.

Dröes, R.M., Meiland, F.J.M., Schmitz, M., Tilburg, W. van (2006). Effect of the Meeting Centers Support Programme on informal carers of people with dementia: Results from a multi-center study. *Aging and Mental Health*, 10(2):112-24.

Dröes RM, Meiland FJM, Schmitz MJ, Vernooij-Dassen MJFJ, Lange J de, Derksen E, Boerema I, Grol RPTM, Tilburg W van. (2003). Implementatie Model Ontmoetingscentra; een onderzoek naar de voorwaarden voor succesvolle landelijke implementatie van ontmoetingscentra voor mensen met dementie en hun verzorgers. Eindrapport maart 2003. VU medical center, Department of Psychiatry: Amsterdam.

Dröes RM, Tilburg W van. (1996). Amélioration du comportement agressif par des activités psychomotrices. *L'Année Gérontologique*, 10: 471-482.

Edwards C, Staniszweska S, Crichton N. (2004). Investigation of the ways in which patients'reports of their satisfaction with healthcare are constructed. *Sociol Health Illn*, 26(2): 159-183.

Finnema EJ, Dröes RM, Ribbe MW, Tilburg W van. (2000). The effects of emotion-oriented approaches in the care for persons suffering from dementia: A review of the literature. *Int. J. Geriatr. Psychiatry*, 15(2): 141-161.

Flint AJ. (1995). Effects of respite care on patients with dementia and their caregivers. *Int. Psychogeriatr.*, 7(4): 505-517.

Forbes DA, Neufeld A. (1997). Strategies to address the methodological challenges of client-satisfaction research in home care. *Can. J. Nurs. Res.*, 29(2): 69-77.

Gaugler JE, Jarrot SE, Zarit SH, Stephens MAP, Townsend A, Greene R. (2003). Adult day service use and reductions in caregiving hours: effect on stress and psychological well-being for dementia caregivers. *Int. J. Geriatr. Psychiatry,* 18: 55-62.

Gerritsen, DL, Dröes RM., Ettema TP, Boelens E, Bos J, Meihuizen L, de Lange J, Schölzel-Dorenbos CJ, Hoogeveen F. (2010). Quality of life in dementia, opinions among people with dementia, their professional caregivers, and in literature]. *Tijdschr Gerontol. Geriatr.*, 41(6): 241-55.

Gibson F. (1994). What can reminiscence contribute to people with dementia? In: *Reminiscence reviewed: evaluations, achievements, perspectives*, Bornat J (ed.). Open University Press: Buckingham, England.

Goffin JJM, Dröes RM, Breebaart E, Mooijaart I, Tilburg W van. (1996). Tevredenheid van de deelnemers over de geïntegreerde ondersteuning. In: Dröes RM. (ed.), Amsterdamse Ontmoetingscentra; een nieuwe vorm van ondersteuning voor mensen met dementie en hun verzorgers. Thesis Publishers: Amsterdam.

Goldberg DP, Hillier VF. (1979). A scaled version of the General Health Questionnaire. *Psychological Medicine*, 9: 139-145.

Hadderingh E, Kootte M, Velde BP te, Kempen GIJM, Breemen WM van den. (1991). De zorg aan thuiswonende dementerende ouderen; een inventariserend casusonderzoek naar knelpunten in de zorg voor dementerende ouderen in de provincie Groningen. Van Denderen: Groningen.

Karlsson I, Båne G, Melin E, Nüth AL, Rybo E. (1985). Mental activation - Brain plasticity. In: *Normal Aging, Alzheimer's Disease and senile dementia*, Gottfries CG (ed.), Editions de l'Université de Bruxelles: Bruxelles.

Kat MG, Jonghe JFM de, Aalten P, Kalisvaart CJ, Dröes RM, Verhey FRJ. (2002). Neuropsychiatric symptoms of dementia: psychometric aspects of the Dutch version of the Neuropsychiatric Inventory (NPI). *Tijdschrift voor Gerontologie en Geriatrie*, 33: 150-155.

Knight BG, Lutzky SM, Macofsky-Urban F. (1993). A meta-analytic review of interventions for caregiver distress: Recommendations for future research. *Gerontologist,* 33(2): 240-248.

Lange J de, Dröes RM, Finnema E and Kooij CH van der. (1999). Aansluiting bij de belevingswereld; Effectieve zorg voor dementerenden. *Alzheimer Magazine*, 12: 16-19.

Lawton MP, Brody EM, Saperstein AR. (1989). A controlled study of respite care service for caregivers of Alzheimer's patients. *Gerontologist,* 29(1): 8-15.

Lewis JR. (1994). Patient views on quality care in general practice: literature review. *Soc. Sci. Med.*, 39(5): 655-670.

Meguro M, Kasai M, Akanuma K, Ishii H, Yamaguchi S, Meguro K. (2008). Comprehensive approach of Donepezil and psychosocial interventions on cognitive function and quality of life for Alzheimer's disease: the Osaki-Tajiri Project. *Age Ageing,* 37:469-473.

Meiland FJM, Dröes RM, Lange J de, Vernooij-Dassen M. (2004). Development of a theoretical model for tracing facilitators and barriers in adaptive implementation of innovative practices in dementia care. *Arch. Gerontol. Geriatr. suppl.* 9: 279-290.

Meiland FJ, Kat MG, van Tilburg W, Jonker C, Dröes RM. (2005). The Emotional Impact of Psychiatric Symptoms in Dementia on Partner Caregivers: Do Caregiver, Patient, and Situation Characteristics Make a Difference? *Alzheimer Dis. Assoc Disord.*,19(4):195-201.

Metitieri T, Zanetti O, Geroldi C, Frisoni GB, De LD, Dello, BM, Bianchetti A, Trabucchi, M. (2001). Reality orientation therapy to delay outcomes of progression in patients with dementia. A retrospective study. *Clin. Rehabil.*,15: 471-478.

Mittelman MS, Ferris SH, Shulman E, Steinberg G, Ambinder A, Mackell JA, Cohen J. (1995). A comprehensive support program: effect on depression in spouse-caregivers of AD patients. *Gerontologist,* 35(6): 792-802.

Mittelman MS, Ferris SH, Shulman E, Steinberg G, Levin, B. (1996). A family intervention to delay nursing home placement of patients with Alzheimer Disease. *JAMA*, 276(21): 1725-1731.

Morris RG, Morris LW, Britton PG. 1989. Social support networks and formal support as factors influencing the psychological adjustment of spouse caregivers of dementia sufferers. *Int. J. Geriat. Psychiatry*, 4: 47-51.

Muskens JB. 1993. Het beloop van dementie; een exploratief longitudinaal onderzoek in de huisartsenpraktijk. Academisch proefschrift, Katholieke Universiteit Nijmegen: Nijmegen.

Osté J, Dröes RM. (2004). Implementatieonderzoek Surinaams Ontmoetingscentrum voor mensen met dementie en hun verzorgers. Afdeling Psychiatrie, VU medisch centrum: Amsterdam.

Pusey H, Richards D. (2001). A systematic review of the effectiveness of psychosocial interventions for carers of people with dementia. *Aging Ment Health*, 5(2): 107-119.

Reisberg B. (1983). The Brief Cognitive Rating Scale and Global Deterioration Scale. In: T. Crook, S. Ferris and C. Barsus (eds). *Assessment in Geriatric psychopharmacology*. Mark Powley Ass Inc: New Canaan (Conn.); 19-35.

Reisberg B, Borenstein J, Salob SP, Ferris SH, Franssen E, Georgotas A. (1987). Behavioral symptoms in Alzheimer's disease: Phenomenology and treatment. *J. Clinical. Psychiat.,* 48(5): 9-15.

Roest HG van der, Meiland FJ, Haaker T, Reitsma E, Wils H, Hout HPJ van, Jonker C, Dröes RM. (2008). Finding the service you need: Human centered design of a Digital Interactive Social Chart in DEMentia Care (DEM-DISC). *The Journal on Information Technology in Healthcare,* 137:210-24.

Sandman PO, Norberg A, Adolfsson R. (1988). Verbal communication and behaviour during meals in five institutionalised patients with Alzheimer-type dementia. *J. Adv. Nurs.*, 13(5): 571-578.

Schultz C. (1991). Dementie onderzoek; een verkennende studie naar de verzorgers van dementerende bejaarden in Amsterdam. Interne publicatie, PCA/Valeriuskliniek: Amsterdam.

Smits CH, de Lange J, Dröes RM, Meiland F, Vernooij-Dassen M, Pot A.M. (2007). Effects of combined intervention programmes for people with dementia living at home and their caregivers: a systematic review. *Int. J. Geriatric. Psychiatry*, 22:1181-1193.

Spector A, Thorgrimsen L, Woods B, Royan L, Davies S, Butterworth M, Orrell M. (2003). Efficacy of an evidence-based cognitive stimulation therapy programme for people with dementia: Randomised Controlled Trial. *British Journal of Psychiatry*, 183: 248-254.

Tadaka E, Kanagawa K. (2004). A randomized controlled trial of a group care program for community-dwelling elderly people with dementia. *Jpn. J. Nurs. Sci.*, 1:19-25.

Teri L, Logsdon RG, Uomoto J, McCurry S.M. (1997). Behavioural treatment of depression in dementia patients: A controlled clinical trial. *J. Gerontol. B. Psychol Sci. Soc. Sci.*, 52: 159-166.

Teunisse S, Haan R de. (1994). Aanpassing van de competentielijst van Vernooij-Dassen (1993). Academic Medical Center; Department of Neurology: Amsterdam.

Toseland RW, Diehl M, Freeman K, Manzanares T, Naleppa M, McCallion P. (1997). The impact of Validation group therapy on nursing home residents with dementia. *J. Appl. Gerontol.,* 16(1): 31-50.

Van Mierlo LD, Van der Roest HG, Meiland FJM, Dröes RM. (2010). Personalized Dementia Care; proven effectiveness of psychosocial interventions in subgroups. *Ageing Res. Rev,* 9(2):163-83. [Epub ahead of print] 2009 Sep 23.

Vernooij-Dassen MJFJ, Lamers C, Bor J, Felling AJA, Grol R. (2000). Prognostic factors of effectiveness of a support program for caregivers of dementia patients. *Int. J. Aging Hum.* Dev, 51(4): 259-274.

Woods RT. (1996). Psychological 'therapies' in dementia. In: *Handbook of the clinical psychology of ageing, Woods RT* (ed.). John Wiley and Sons Ltd: Chichester, England.

Woods RT. (2001). Discovering the person with Alzheimer's disease: cognitive, emotional and behavioural aspects. *Aging Ment Health*, 5(suppl 1): S7-16.

Zarit SH, Gaugler JE, Jarrot SE. (1999). Useful services for families: Research findings and directions. *Int. J. Geriatr. Psychiatry*, 14: 165-181.

In: Non-Pharmacological Therapies ...
Editor: Elisabetta Farina

ISBN: 978-1-63321-860-4

Chapter 5

Pilot Study Protocol of an Educational Intervention for Caregivers of People with Psychological and Behavioral Symptoms Due to Dementia*

S. F. Vitali[1], C. Cutaia[2] and R. Vaccaro[2]
[1]C. Golgi Geriatric Institute Abbiategrasso (MI) Italy
[2]Golgi Cenci Foundation Abbiategrasso (MI) Italy

Abstract

The purpose of the study is to describe an educational program for caregivers of people with dementia and behavioral-psychological symptoms (BPSD), admitted to the Special Care Unit (SCU) of our Institute for a temporary stay. The prosthetic approach used in the SCU considers informal caregivers (families) as partner of the formal ones (staff) in building up the program of care.

The intervention is aimed at extending to the caregivers an interpretative approach to the BPSD, and at sharing with them the results of a systematic approach used from the staff to understand the possible causes of these symptoms.

The core of the intervention is based first on training the family in learning ABC (antecedents-behavior-consequences) approach to assess and monitor the PWD (person with dementia) behaviors, then on training and supporting caregivers to apply the suggested interventions.

At the same time caregiving issues appearing during the period of their stay in the unit are addressed in a therapeutically alliance with the family. The hypothesis we assume is that this practice will be able to enhance caregivers ability to manage critical situation in the care process. Outcome measures will be caregivers self efficacy and stress measures.

---

* Part of this paper has been showed as an oral presentation in the "Second course on Non-pharmacological Therapies in Dementia: focus on the caregiver", Milan, October, 15, 2011.

Keywords: Alzheimer's disease, dementia, Behavior and Psychological Symptoms of Dementia (BPSD), interpretative approach, caregiving self-efficacy and stress, prosthetic approach

Introduction

Dementia is associated with progressive cognitive and functional disability, as well with a high prevalence of behavioral and psychological symptoms (BPSD), often resulting in suffering for patient and caregivers, loss of quality of life, premature institutionalization, increased cost of care. The Prosthetic Approach, derived from Gentle Care by Moyra Jones, (Guaita A et al.2011; Jones M. 1996) used in our Special Care Unit (SCU) (Guaita 2000) considers most BPSD of dementia as a possible language used by the person with dementia to communicate needs or discomfort that the person is not able to express differently, in relation to the cognitive deficits due to neurodegeneration. Staff in the SCU refers to the bio-psycho-social framework to look for possible causes of BPSD and uses the P-I-E-C-E-S approach (Le Clair K, 2008-see later for the meaning of the acronimous) to promote the understanding of PWD complex physical, cognitive/affective health needs and associated behavioral issues. In a previous study (Colombo M., Vitali S. 2007) we have demonstrated the improvement of BPSD in a sample of 214 PWD during the stay in the SCU.

These improvements followed trajectories that were consistent with baseline groupings, by factor analysis. The prosthetic approach looks at PWD informal caregivers both as partner of the individual care program and as a target for specific educational intervention when dysfunctional behaviors in the care routine or the excessive care burden impact negatively on the PWD and create distress in the caregiver himself. There have been studies that show differences between the ways of adapting to the caregiver role (Anhelsen et al.1995). The risk of developing psychological distress with depression and anxiety was also confirmed in a previous study on caregivers of PWD admitted in our SCU. (Malnati, M. et al., 2009)

Purpose of the Study-Intervention

Previous studies on educational program and care interventions in community context have demonstrated some results on reducing caregivers' distress.(Brodaty H. et al. 2003, Burns R. et al. ,2003, Mittelman MS, et al. 2004). The hypothesis we assume is that the more we are able to empower the caregiver in understanding the dementia process and the relation between biological, psychological, interpersonal and social aspects in generating BPSD, while addressing at the same time the emerging caregiving issues, the more the caregiver can control and manage critical situation in the care process. The temporary stay of PWD in the SCU gives staff and families a unique opportunity to work together in a therapeutically alliance for a considerable period of time (about two months).

Study aims are the following:

- to extend to the family caregivers an interpretative approach to the BPSD while the PWD is in-patient and to share with the family the results of a systematic approach used from the staff to understand the possible causes of the BPSD (PIECES approach)

- To guide the family in learning and using the ABC approach (Smith M. et al. 2005; Moniz Cook E. D. et al 2009) to assess and monitor the PWD behavior
- To train and to support family caregivers to apply and monitor interventions
- To evaluate the impact of such a process on family caregivers self-efficacy and personal control in managing BPSD
- To evaluate the impact of such an approach on family caregivers stress levels

The ABC approach in understanding and responding to behavior in PWD is a well known psychological paradigm targeted at describing the behavior (B) that causes distress to the patient and or to the caregiver, identifying the antecedents(A's), and the consequences (C's) of the behavior itself. The identification of the function of a specific behavior for that specific individual (why here, why now, what set it off) let caregivers derive some hypothesis-driven non pharmacological interventions. Training and supporting family and staff caregivers to apply and monitor interventions that are considered functional to reduce PWD distress is the conclusive part of the intervention.

In PIECES framework the first three letters P-I-E represent the individual Physical-Intellectual and Emotional health, the C are the capabilities, the E-S represent the environment that the individual interacts with and the personal Social self (values, spirituality etc). Understanding P-I-E issues, assessing the Capabilities and evaluating the context of life and care, E-S, is crucial to know the PWD needs we are facing at, to answer properly and consequently to readdress behavior.

Methodology

The study is intended to evaluate 25 caregiver without a control group to test the validity of the protocol. The inclusion criteria are:

- Being caregivers of PWD with BPSD
- Being the principal caregiver
- Having the willingness to participate to meetings with the team work

Assessment of the PWD

- Physical: diagnosis (standardized criteria NINCS-ADRDA-McKhann G. et al 1984); Comorbidities (CIRS- Cumulative Illness Rating Scale-Parmalee PA et al, 1995); queries delirium; pain and discomfort, medications, conducted by medical staff
- Intellectual: MMSE (Mini Mental State Examination- Folstein MF et al 1975) and Neuropsychological evaluation, speech evaluation, insight (CIRS- Clinical Insight Rating Scale Ott BR et al. 1996), staging (CDR- Clinical Dementia Rating Hughs 1982) conducted by medical-psychological and speech therapy staff

- Emotional: mood, anxiety and psychotic disorders by NPI (Neuropsychiatric Inventory-Cummings J. et al 1994) items and psychological evaluation, conducted by medical and psychological staff
- Capabilities: functional assessment, deficits and strengths, Lawton Instrumental Activities -Lawton and Brody 1969, Barthel Index- Shah S. et al1989, Tinetti M. gait and balance-Tinetti 1986 , Assessment Movement and Process Skills (AMPS modified) Fisher AG. 1997 for procedural aspects, MOVI modified- Cunningham Pierogrossi J. 2006 conducted by rehabilitation staff. MOVI is a an occupational approach based on psychological concepts. It aims to stress the emotional aspects of the relationship between the OT and the PWD, as well as the emotional contents of the occupational intervention itself.
- Environment: ability to read the context, level or type of stimulation, care routine, physical space (everyone's job)
- Social: Life story, life accomplishments, relationships of family, lifelong coping strategies. The interview is conducted by the Occupational Therapist (OT)

Assessment of the Family Caregiver by the Psychologist

- Needs analysis: semi-structured interview adapted from Pearlin LI. et al 1990 and Paton J. et al.2004, before and after the intervention The interview explores the self-perception of the caregiver (items derived from Perlin' Scale, 1990), caregivers' understanding of the causes of behaviors they find problematic (items derived from Paton 2004) and the quality of relationship with PWD.
- Family strategies in practical situations: multiple choice questionnaire before and after the intervention The questionnaire describes the common caregiver responses to the problem behaviors (as delusions, resistive and aggressive behaviors and aberrant motor behavior) that are the most troubling according clinical experience in our Special Care Unit.
- Stress level: Zarit Burden Interview (Chattat R. et al 2010) self administered before and after the intervention

Intervention Description

Family caregivers meet three times the medical doctor and the psychologist, two times the occupational therapist .The doctor and the OT meet the family caregivers at first, share with the team in a weekly scheduled meeting the results of the evaluation, report the situations that might need the psychologist intervention.

Meetings with the Psychologist

During the first meeting the psychologist leads the caregiver through needs analysis aimed to understand the following issues:

- Behaviors that are more distressing
- Caregiver's insight about PWD behavior
- Caregiver's approach to the distressing behavior
- Caregiver's emotional reaction during the distressing behavior
- Pre-morbid relationship and the change trough the progression of the disease
- Caregiver's insight about the disease
- Caregiver's insight about self efficacy and control

Then the psychologist evaluates family strategies in practical situations using the multiple choice questionnaire, evaluates the stress level through self administered Zarit Burden Interview and finally introduces the ABC elements.

The second meeting is structured in two moments: half an hour session with a direct observation of the interaction between the PWD and the caregiver during the care routine. One hour session is then dedicated to focus on the ABC approach in relation to issues that have come out from the direct observation and on similar situations that could trigger BPSD at home.

A third and conclusive meeting is addressed to caregivers description of the strategies applied with the PWD, to discussion about what have worked and what not, to reconsidering realistic expectation and, if necessary, to rephrasing the ABC approach. The psychologist's final evaluation closes the meeting.

Meetings with the Doctor

First meeting takes place at the admission of the PWD, to collect clinical history and to make a first context analysis following PIECES framework. A second meeting is scheduled after two weeks for the feedback on the team evaluation results. A third meeting is conducted one week before the discharge for a feedback on the conclusive results and therapeutic suggestions.

Meeting with OT

A first meeting takes place before the admission with an evaluation of PWD home routine, communication ability, sensory impairment, problem with the environment. The caregiver is asked to fill the biography form and to bring familiar objects to personalize the room. One week before the discharge, another meeting takes place to present and discuss with family the routine's meaningful program shaped during PWD stay in the unit. If necessary, suggestions about environment modification at home to solve specific problem (safety and security, function and activity, access and mobility) are given.Results will be registered and elaborated with SPSS11.0. Descriptive statistics of the sample will be provided: PWD cognitive and functional profiles, frequency of the BPSD, behaviors that are judged more distressing by the carers. Variance analysis of burden, caregivers' attitudes, insight, auto efficacy and control will be considered. Burden, caregivers attitudes, insight, auto efficacy and control will be analyzed with parametric or non parametric statistical tests when appropriate. Preliminary ResultsFrom February to October 2011, thirteen caregivers attended the study, but three of them dropped out after the first meeting with the psychologist. Nine caregivers completed the educational program.

The group is too small to allow drawing definitive conclusions about the results of the intervention; so we report preliminary results on group features. The first meeting with the psychologist was carried out within seven days, after a doctor's warning. . Seven caregivers were women (four daughters and three wives); six caregivers were men (four sons and two husbands). The most frequent caregivers' works were white collar and housewife.

Five PWD were affected by Alzheimer disease, three by Vascular dementia and five by other kind of dementia.

a) Most Relevant Reported Behavioral Problems and Related Caregivers' Attributions

- Delusions and verbal aggression (cussing, swearing, and raising the voice) were described as the most upsetting behaviors by caregivers. Nine of them identify as cause of these behaviors a psychiatric or organic disease.
- Verbal repetition was referred by some caregivers as the principal problem although isn't considered a BPSD by literature.
- Memory deficit is misinterpreted: only five caregivers charged this deficit to dementia, the other ones attributed it to psychological or medical problems.
- Most of caregivers only partially understood the diagnosis, even if they are aware of disease progression.
- Patients were considered unable to control actively their own disturbed behaviors

b) Caregiver's Reaction to Problematic Behaviors

Caregiver's reactions towards BPSD were mostly inefficacy interventions as blaming or trying to convince the patient to change their behavior. In other cases the inefficacy reaction was a closing behavior as crying or being indifferent, cold or silent

c) Caregivers' Emotional Feelings and Influence of the Pre-Morbid Quality of the Relationship

Most of the caregivers felt a negative emotion (frustration) as a consequence of patients' problematic behaviors. Ten of the thirteen caregivers felt role captivity: they wished to leave the patient or to withdraw into themselves. In seven of the cases the pre-morbid quality relation with the patient was negative: mostly conflictual, cold or devaluing. Most of the caregivers referred that dementia brought a worsening of the relationship with the PWD. In other cases they reported that the negative relationship was unchanged.

d) Autoefficacy and Distress

All caregivers had self-confidence and felt quite able to manage problems related to problematic behaviors, even if they had doubts about their auto-efficacy. The analysis of the Zarit Burden Interview showed a qualitative positive trend in caregiver's stress reduction, while a first analysis of the multiple choice questionnaire showed an improvement in the use of the effective strategies only in four of the cases.

Conclusion

Preliminary data we collected show that caregivers have acquired a knowledge about some aspects of the disease, such as its progression and the fact that it causes a lack of control on behavior, but they have not understood neither the relationship between the disease pathology and the behavioral changes, nor the interaction between the environmental distress and the appearance of dysfunctional behaviors. They consider BPSD as an expression of conflicts in personal relationship. In this sample most caregivers referred a longstanding negative relationship with PWD. The relational patterns and the dysfunctional communication continue to be acted out in the present. These results confirm what reported in the literature about the importance of the stable caregiver characteristics as a determinant of the way used in managing the patients (de Vugt M, 2004). The caregivers had self-confidence and felt quite able to manage problems related to behaviors, even if they had doubts about their auto efficacy. This sense of inefficacy can be explained by the poor understanding of the situation, that is an important mediator of psychological well-being for caregivers (Hepburn K, et al 2001) The errors of attribution and the lack of auto efficacy were associated with negative emotion and role captivity. The focus on the ABC approach in relation to issues that have come out from the direct observation helped caregivers to become aware about that and allowed learning through experience. Family caregivers are partners of the person's centered care program because of their knowledge about PWD needs but at the same time they are the target of our therapeutic intervention. Their attitude of care has great influence on PWD behavior and they will continue to take care of the PWD after the discharge. Longstanding personality traits and quality of the caregiver – PWD emotional relationship have not only the potential to exacerbate or to alleviate the occurrence and the impact of BPSD but also the ability to affect the learning of the ABC approach. The counseling from the psychologist is an opportunity to make the caregiver aware about that and to personalize the learning process. The development of a common vision, a common language and a common approach to BPSD and to the complex needs of the PWD, is the core of the therapeutic alliance between staff and family caregivers, which is a cornerstone in the prosthetic approach .The final results of our study will allow to appreciate whether this kind of intervention has the potential to reduce problematic behavioral problems at home and whether a larger study deserves to be planned in order to definitively confirm the efficacy of the prosthetic approach.

References

Anhelsen, C.S., Pearlin, L.I., Zarit, S.H., Witlach, C.J. (1995) Profiles in caregiving: the unexpected career. San Diego Academic Press.

Brodaty,H. Green.A, 2003). A Meta-analysis of psychosocial interventions for caregivers of people with dementia. *J. Am. Geriatr. Soc.,* 51 657–664.

Burns, R. Nichols, L. et al. (2003) Primary care interventions for dementia caregivers: 2-year outcomes from the REACH study. *The Gerontologist,* 43, 547-557.

Cunningham Pierogrossi, J. (2006) Essere nel fare- Introduzione alla terapia occupazionale. Firenze Franco Angeli Chattat, R., Cortesi Izzicupo, F., Del Re, ML., Sgarbi, C., Fabbo,

A., Bergonzini E.(2010) The Italian version of the Zarit Burden Interview: a validation study. *Int. Psychogeriatr.* 16,1-9.

Colombo, M., Vitali, SF., Cairati, M., Vaccaro, R., Andreoni, G., Guaita, A.(2007) Behavioral and Psychotic Simptoms of Dementia (BPSD) Improvements in a Special Care Unit : A factor Analysis.*Arch. Geronthol. Geriatr.* Suppl 1, 113-120.

Cummings, J., Mega, M., Gray, K., et al.(1994) The Neuropsychiatric Inventory: Comprehensive assessment of psychopathology in dementia. *Neurology*, 44, 2308-2314.

De Vugt M.E., Stevens F., Aalten P., Lousberg R., Jaspers N., Winkens I., Jolles J., Verhey F.R.J., (2004) Do caregiver management strategies influence patient behaviour in dementia? *Int. J. Geriatr. Psychiatry*, 19, 85-92.

Fisher, A.G., (1997) Assessment of Motor and Process Skills. 2nd ed. Fort Collins, CO: Three Star Press.

Folstein. MF., Folstein. SE., McHugh, PR. (1975) Mini-mental state. A practical method for grading he cognitive state of patients for the clinician. *Journal of Psychiatric Research, 12 (3), 189–98.*

Guaita, A., Jones, M. (2011) A "Prosthetic" Approach for individual with dementia *JAMA,* 35, 402-403.

Guaita, A. (2000) The Special Care Units for people with Alzheimer's disease and other dementia syndromes indicator of the quality of the intervention. *Giorn. Gerontol*, 48, 42-47.

Gitlin, Laura N. et al. (2010) Targeting and Managing Behavioral Symptoms in Individuals with Dementia: A Randomized trial of a non Pharmacological intervention. *J. Am. Ger. Soc.,* 58,1465-1474.

Hepburn K.W., Tornatore J, Center B., Ostwald S.W, (2001) Dementia family caregiver training: affecting beliefs about caregiving and caregivers outcomes, *JAGS*, 49, 450-457.

Hughes, CP., et al. (1982) A new clinical scale for the staging of Dementia. *Br. J. Psychiatry,140, 566-572.*

Jones, M., Guaita, A., Vitali, SF., et al (1996) Gentle Care: a new prosthetic approach to the care of demented elderly people. The Lancet Conference: The Challenge of the dementias. Edimburgh UK April 25-26 p89 (abstract only).

Malnati, M., Vaccaro,R., Cutaia, C., Colombo, M., D'Angelo, R., Guaita, A., Procino, G., Vitali, S.F.(2009) Analisi di correlati psicologici e biologici dello stress in familiari di persone con e senza demenza temporaneamente ricoverate. Giornale di gerontologia, 8,478.

McKhann, G., Drachman, D., Folstein, M., Katzman, R., Price, D., Stadlan, EM. (1984) Clinical Diagnosis of Alzheimer's Disease. Report of the NINCDS-ADRDA Work Group. *Neurology,* 34, 934-943.

Mittelman, MS., Roth, DL., Coon, DW., et al (2004) Sustained benefit of supportive intervention for depressive symptoms in Alzheimer's caregivers. *Am. J. Psychiatry,* 161, 850–856.

Monitz Cook, ED., DeVugt. M., Verhey F., James, I. (2009) Functional analysis-based interventions for challanging behavior in dementia. (protocol) *The Cochrane Library,* Issue 1.

Morris, J.C., (1993) The Clinical Dementia Rating (CDR): Current version and scoring rules. *Neurology,* 43, 2412-2414.

Ott, BR., Lafleche, G., et al. (1996) Impaired Awareness of deficits in Alzheimer's disease. *Alzh. Dis. Ass. Disorders* ,10, 68-76.

Parmalee, PA., Thuras, PD., Lawton, MP. (1995) Validation of cumulative Illness Rating Scale in a residential geriatric population. *J. Am. Geriatr. Soc.*, 43,130-137.

Paton, J., Johnston, K., Katona, C., Livingston, G., (2004) What causes problems in Alzheimer's disease : attributions by caregivers. A qualitative study. *Intern. J. of Geriatr. Psychiatry,* 19,527-37.

Pearlin, LI., et al (1990) Caregiving and The Stress Process: An overview of Concepts and Mesaures. *The Gerontologist,* 30, n°5.

Smith, M., Buckwalter, K. (2005) Back to A-B-C's. Understanding and responding to behavioural Symptoms in dementia. Revised from Acting Up and Acting Out: Assessment and Management of Aggressive and Acting out Behavior. *The Geriatric Mental Health Training Series for the Hartford Center of Geriatric Nursing Excellence, College of Nursing, University of Iowa.*

Stolee , P., McCainey, CA., Hillier, LM., Harris, D., Hamilton, P., Kessler, L., Madsen, V., Le Clair, K., (2009) Sustained Transfer of Knowledge to Practice in Long-Term Care: Facilitators and Barriers of a Mental Health Learning Initiative, *Gerontology and Geriatrics Education,* 30, 1-20.

Shah, S., Vanclay, F., Cooper, B., (1989) Improving the Sensivity of Barthel Index for stroke rehabilitation. *J.Clin.Epidemiol.*,42,703-709.

Tinetti, M., (1986) Performance-oriented assessment of mobility problems in elderly patient. *J. Am. Geriatr. Soc.* 34, 119 – 136.

In: Non-Pharmacological Therapies ...
Editor: Elisabetta Farina

ISBN: 978-1-63321-860-4

Chapter 6

The Additional Contribution of Combination of Pharmacological Therapy and Cognitive Stimulation in Alzheimer's Disease: Review of the Literature

Maria Cotelli, Rosa Manenti and Orazio Zanetti
IRCCS Psychiatry, Centro San Giovanni di Dio - Fatebenefratelli Brescia, Italy

Abstract

Alzheimer's disease (AD) is a progressive disorder that impacts several cognitive functions. However, some aspects of cognitive function are preserved until later in the disease and can therefore be the targets of specific interventions. The rehabilitation of cognitive function disorders represents an expanding area of neurological rehabilitation and it has recently attracted growing political, social and ethical attention. Here we review the efficacy of combining cognitive stimulation and cholinesterase inhibitors. Generally, all the studies reported in this review have compared the combined treatment with pharmacological intervention alone. Further studies should clarify the potential role of the combined cognitive-pharmacological treatment in AD persons with dementias care. In the meantime, the findings of the studies reviewed in this paper suggest that cognitive rehabilitation should be an essential part of dementia treatment, along with anti-dementia drugs.

Keywords: Alzheimer's disease (AD), combined cognitive-pharmacological treatment, rehabilitation of cognitive function disorders

Alzheimer's Disease (AD) is the most common cause of dementia and results in a slowly progressive impairment of cognitive functions. Behavioural and functional impairment following AD constitutes one of the major causes of disability worldwide. Moreover, it has a significant impact on the lives of affected individuals and on quality of life of their families.

It is now well known the limited effectiveness of pharmacological treatments that have symptomatic effect in only a minority portion of persons with dementia (donepezil, rivastigmine, galantamine and memantine). Therefore non-pharmacological interventions in AD have gained attention in recent years and there are currently many different approaches under study, ranging from multi-strategy approaches to cognitive training (Buschert, Bokde, and Hampel, 2010; Olazaran et al., 2010). Non-pharmacological interventions may play a role in planning multidimensional models for dementia care, treating the cognitive, functional, behavioural and affective aspects of dementia (Cotelli, Calabria, and Zanetti, 2006). Furthermore, some studies have compared pharmacological interventions both with cognitive treatments and with the combination of these two treatments, revealing that cognitive approaches (cognitive training, cognitive rehabilitation and Reality Orientation Therapy) could be an effective complementary tool in the treatment of cognitive deficits in these persons with dementia.

This paper describes the main studies that compared the efficacy in persons with dementia of pharmacological treatment combined with cognitive stimulation vs. pharmacological treatment alone (Table 1). The primary criterion for inclusion in this review was that studies included a control group with a drug only treatment in order to highlight the additional gain induced by the combined treatment. Memantine treatment has not been considered due to the lack of studies.

In two subsequent studies, Requena et al. (2004; 2006) described persons with a diagnosis of AD divided in four subgroups according to the treatment they received: a) combined pharmacological and cognitive treatment, b) only pharmacological intervention, c) only cognitive stimulation and d) no treatment at all. Thus, these authors considered all possible comparisons, including the combined treatment, cognitive training alone and no treatment. This is an important issue, which allowed both evaluation of the effects induced by cognitive rehabilitation alone and direct comparison of the two treatments (cognitive or pharmacological) applied separately. Cognitive stimulation treatment comprised different areas of stimulation: orientation, bodily awareness, family and society, caring for oneself, reminiscing, household activities, animals, people and things. Each session lasted 45 min and sessions were held 5 days a week for 12 months (Requena et al., 2004). Requena et al. (2006) evaluated the efficacy of those treatments administered over the course of two years. The authors proposed cognitive evaluation before the beginning of the treatment and after 12 months in both studies, whereas cognitive evaluation was also performed after 24 months in the second study. In the first study (Requena et al., 2004), 86 AD persons were included and the results showed that subjects receiving the combined treatment improved in terms of cognitive processes compared to the subjects who received drug treatment alone and those who received no treatment. In addition, the persons with dementia that received only cognitive stimulation as opposed to those who did not receive any treatment achieved better results on cognitive tests.

Table 1. studies that compared the efficacy in persons with dementia of pharmacological treatment combined with cognitive stimulation vs. pharmacological treatment alone

Study	Methods	N° of patients	Cholinesterase inhibitors (ChEI)	Rehabilitation Intervention (Reh)	Treatment duration (weeks)	Asse-ssments (weeks)	Outcome measures	Results
Requena et al., 2004	Group 1: Reh+ChEI Group 2: ChEI Group 3: Reh Group 4: none	86	Donepezil, 5 mg/day for the first 5 weeks and 10 mg/day thereafter	Cognitive stimulation (seven areas of stimulation). 5 days a week + 2 days a week in-home treatment, 45 minutes a day.	52	52	MMSE, ADAS-cog, GDS, FAST	Group 1: improvement in MMSE, ADAS-cog and FAST Group 2: decline in MMSE, ADAS-cog and FAST Group 3: improvement in MMSE, ADAS-cog, GDS and FAST Group 4: decline in MMSE, ADAS-cog and FAST and improvement in GDS.
Chapman et al., 2004	Group 1: Reh+ChEI Group 2: ChEI	54	Donepezil	Cognitive-Communication program, 1 days a week, 90 minutes a day	8	8, 32, 52	MMSE, ADAS-cog, NPI, Composite of Discourse, TFLS, CIBIC, QOL	Group 1: decline in TFLS, less than Group 2, improvement in CIBIC Group 2: decline in MMSE, Composite of Discourse, TFLS, NPI irritability subscale
Onder et al., 2005	Group 1: Reh+ChEI Group 2: ChEI	156	Donepezil, 5 mg/day (69 patients) or 10 mg/day (87 patients)	In-home ROT by the caregiver, 3 days a week, 30 minutes a day	25	25	MMSE, ADAS-cog, Barthel index, IADL, NPI. Caregiver assessment: HRSD, HRSA, SF-36, CBI	Group 1: improvement in MMSE and ADAS-cog Group 2: decline in MMSE and ADAS-cog
Bottino et al., 2005	Group 1: Reh+ChEI Group 2: ChEI	13	Rivastigmine, 6 mg/day (8 patients) or 9 mg/day (3 patients) or 12 mg/day (2 patients)	Cognitive Stimulation, 1 day a week, 90 minutes a day	25	25	MMSE, ADAS-cog, IADL, FDS, BDS, CDR, WAIS subtests, VF AND BNT. Caregiver assessment: MADRS, HRSA,	Group 1: improvement in MMSE and BDS Group 2: no changes
Requena et al., 2006	Group 1: Reh+ChEI Group 2: ChEI Group 3: Reh Group 4: none	78	Donepezil, 5 mg/day for the first 5 weeks and 10 mg/day thereafter	Cognitive stimulation (Seven areas of stimulation). 5 days a week + 1 day in-home training, 45 minutes a day	104	52; 104	MMSE, ADAS-cog, GDS, FAST	Group 1: improvement in ADAS-cog, GDS at 52 weeks and in GDS at 104 weeks Group 2: decline in MMSE, ADAS-cog and FAST at 52 weeks and at 104 weeks; improvement in GDS only at 52 weeks; Group 3: improvement in MMSE, ADAS-cog and FAST at 52 weeks; Group 4: decline in MMSE, ADAS-cog and FAST at 52 and 104 weeks; improvement in GDS at 52 and 104 weeks.

Table 1. (Continued)

Study	Methods	No of patients	Cholinesterase inhibitors (ChEI)	Rehabilitation (Reh) Intervention	Treatment duration (weeks)	Asse-ssments (weeks)	Outcome measures	Results
Tarraga et al., 2006	Group 1: Reh+PSY+ChEI Group 2: PSY+ChEI Group 3: ChEI	43	ChEI	Interactive multimedia internet-based system approach 3 days a week for 15 (first 24 sessions), 20 (sessions 25-28), or 25 (sessions 29-72) minutes. Integrated Psychostimulation Program 480 minutes a day, 5 days a week.	24	12; 24	MMSE, ADAS-cog, SKT, BNT, verbal fluency, story recall from the RBMT, RDRS, GDS	Group 1: better than Group 3 in ADAS-cog and MMSE at 12 and 24 weeks; Group 2: better than Group 3 in ADAS-cog and MMSE at 12 weeks and only in MMSE at 24 weeks.
Matsuda, 2007	Group 1: Reh+ChEI Group 2: ChEI	30	Donepezil, 5 mg/day	Cognitive stimulation, 60 minutes a day, 1 day a week for the first 8 sessions and 1 each two weeks for the subsequent sessions.	52	52	MMSE	Group 1: no changes Group 2: decline in MMSE
Giordano et al., 2010	Group 1: Reh+ChEI Group 2: ChEI	100	Donepezil, 5 mg/day	Physical reactivation (15 minutes) + ROT (45 minutes). 6 days a week +1 day a week in-home training	3 + 9 in-home training	3; 9	MMSE, ADAS-cog, ADL, IADL, PPT	Group 1: improvement in MMSE, ADAS-cog and PPT at 3 weeks; improvement in MMSE at 9 weeks Group 2: improvement in PPT
Matsuda et al., 2010	Group 1: Reh+ChEI Group 2: ChEI	49	Donepezil	Cognitive stimulation, 30 minutes a day, 1 day a week.	7	7	MMSE, HDS-R	Group 1: improvement in HDS-R Group 2: no changes

Cognitive subscale of the Alzheimer's Disease Assessment Scale: ADAS-cog; Backward Digit Span: BDS; Caregiver Burden Inventory: CBI; Boston Naming Test: BNT; Cholinesterase Inhibitors: ChEI; Clinical Dementia Rating Scale: CDR; Clinical Interview-Based Impression of Change: CIBIC; overall deterioration scale: FAST; Forward Digit Span: FDS; Fuld Object Memory Evaluation: FOME; Geriatric Depression Scale: GDS; Hasegawa's Dementia Scale-Revised: HDS-R; Hamilton Rating Scale for Depression: HRSD; Hamilton Rating Scale for Anxiety: HRSA; Instrumental Activities of Daily Living: IADL; Activities of Daily Living: ADL; Montgomery-Asberg Depression Rating Scale: MADRS; Mini-Mental State Examination: MMSE; Neuropsychiatric Inventory: NPI; Reality Orientation Therapy: ROT; Physical Performance Test: PPT; Quality of Life Questionnaire: QOL; Rapid Disability Rating Scale: RDRS; Rivermead Behavioural Memory Test: RBMT; Short-Form General Health Survey: SF-36; Syndrom Kurztest Task: SKT; Texas Functional Living Scale: TFLS; Trail Making Test: TMT; Verbal Fluency: VF; Wechsler Adult Intelligence Scale: WAIS.

To verify the effectiveness of combined treatment over two years with the same group of persons with dementia used in the previous study, Requena et al. (2006) included 78 AD persons treated for 24 months. The results confirmed the previous investigation: cognitive and combined treatment improved persons with dementia' performance throughout the first year. However, the authors showed that, at the 2-years follow-up, all groups deteriorated. The data reported in these studies indicated that cognitive stimulation combined with pharmacological treatment leads to considerable improvements in these persons with dementia. With regard to long-term effects, the authors suggested that cognitive deterioration cannot be stopped, even after 2 years of treatment, even if deterioration is greater and its progress is faster in persons with dementia not receiving any treatment at all.

In both the Requena's group studies no differences between combined treatment and cognitive stimulation have been shown. This makes difficult to clarify the additional gains due to the combined treatment as compared to the cognitive treatment.

Chapman and co-worker (Chapman et al., 2004) in a randomized study evaluated the combined effect of a cognitive-communication program plus a cholinesterase inhibitor as compared with pharmacological treatment alone. The stimulation program consisted of 12 hours of intervention over on 8-weeks period and involved participated discussions requiring homework, interactive session about AD, and discussions using salient life stories. This study revealed benefits of cholinesterase inhibitor-plus-stimulation group in the areas of discourse abilities, functional abilities, emotional symptoms, and overall global performance. These gains have been highlighted comparing the combined treatment group with the pharmacological treatment group. An additional group of persons with dementia treated with the cognitive-communication program alone would have allowed also the investigation of the benefits of the combined treatment compared to cognitive-communication program.

Some studies investigated the effects on cognitive function of a home-based program of Reality Orientation Therapy (ROT) provided by caregivers and applied during pharmacological intervention by comparing this combined treatment with one treatment alone.

ROT is the only established intervention supported by randomised clinical studies that improves cognition and behaviour in persons with mild to moderate dementia (National Institute for Health and Clinical Excellence, 2006; Spector et al., 2004). The major aim of ROT is to increase persons with dementia's orientation to time, place and persons. A Cochrane review (Spector et al., 2004) concluded that ROT should be considered, together with cholinesterase inhibitors, as part of a more general dementia care program.

In a study by Onder et al. (2005), the researchers randomly assigned 79 out of 156 persons with dementia treated with cholinesterase inhibitors to receive ROT treatment. Caregivers of the treatment group were trained to offer the program at home 3 days a week, 30 min/day, for 25 consecutive weeks. The persons with dementia that received the combined treatment showed a slight improvement in the Mini-Mental State Examination [MMSE, (Folstein, Folstein, and McHugh, 1975)] and in the cognitive subscale of the Alzheimer's Disease Assessment Scale [ADAS-cog, (Rosen, Mohs, and Davis, 1984)], in contrast to a decline in the control group that received only pharmacological treatment. The intervention had an equal effect on cognition in those with mild and moderate dementia. Conversely, no differences in behavioural or functional outcomes were observed between the two groups. The authors concluded that reality orientation enhances the effects of pharmacological treatment on cognition in Alzheimer's disease. The results of this interesting study have highlighted the benefits of the combined treatment group as compared to the pharmacological treatment alone group. An additional control group of persons with dementia treated with ROT alone would have allowed the investigation of the benefits of the combined treatment. In a study of Bottino and collegues (Bottino et al., 2005) the researchers studied the efficacy of cognitive rehabilitation combined with cholinesterase inhibitor treatment compared with cholinesterase inhibitor treatment alone in persons with Alzheimer's disease and their relatives. Thirteen persons with mild Alzheimer's disease treated with cholinesterase inhibitors (6-12 mg/day) for more than two months were included. Before and after the treatment persons with dementia were assessed through cognitive tests, activities of daily living scale, neuropsychological battery and scales to evaluate caregivers' depressive and anxiety symptoms. Six persons with dementia were randomized to a combined treatment group and seven persons with dementia to a control group and followed up for five months. The cognitive rehabilitation consisted in 90-minutes group sessions, once a week for five months designed to stimulate persons with dementia's cognitive functions and to enhance daily living and social interaction. At the end of the five months the two AD persons groups were significantly different in Mini-Mental State Examination (MMSE) scores and in backward digit span scores with better results in the combined treatment group than in the control group. The authors concluded that cognitive rehabilitation associated with cholinesterase inhibitors treatment can potentially be useful to stabilize or improve cognitive and functional performance of persons with mild Alzheimer's disease (Bottino et al., 2005). The main limitation of this study is the small sample used. Subsequently, Tarraga et al. (2006) evaluated the effect of an interactive multimedia internet-based system (IMIS) as adjunct to cholinesterase inhibitor therapy and a integrated psychostimulation program (IPP). Forty-six AD persons with dementia were randomly assigned to three groups: 15 participated in the internet-based system plus an integrated psychostimulation program and drug therapy; 16 underwent only integrated psychostimulation program sessions and drug therapy; and 12 received only pharmacological therapy. The internet-based system was conducted using an interactive multi-media tool that included several stimulation programs (attention, calculation, gnosis, language, memory and orientation), whereas the Integrated Psychostimulation Program consisted mainly in reinforcement of the instrumental activities of daily living. Cognitive evaluation was conducted before the beginning of the treatment and after 12 and 24 weeks of treatment. This study showed that both the Integrated Psychostimulation Program and computer-based therapy improved cognition (ADAS-Cog and MMSE) in subjects treated with a stable dose of cholinesterase inhibitor therapy compared to those who were treated only with the drug. In addition, the computer-based program provided an improvement above and beyond that seen with the Integrated Psychostimulation Program, with the improvement lasting 24 weeks. The authors suggested that although both behavioural treatments improved cognition in AD persons more than did pharmacological treatment alone. In addition, the combination of all treatments provided a long-lasting improvement and is therefore recommended. This study demonstrated that it is possible to augment the effects of drugs using non-pharmacological treatment. The inclusion of larger samples and the addiction of a group of persons with dementia treated with IMIS and cholinesterase inhibitor therapy would help to clarify the additional benefits provided by IMIS and IPP compared to the effects of drugs.

Matsuda et al. (2007) evaluated the effect of cognitive stimulation therapy (CST) combined with pharmacological treatment on the progression of cognitive decline among AD persons. CST used by the authors involves guided practice on a set of standard tasks designed to reflect particular cognitive functions and is offered through individual or group sessions, or facilitated by family members with support from therapists. The authors compared the cognitive performance of 17 AD persons treated with 1-year cognitive stimulation plus cholinesterase inhibitors therapy to 13 AD persons treated with pharmacological treatment alone. Persons with dementia in the combined group received pharmacological treatment and participated in about 20 one-hour CST sessions during one year. The first eight sessions were carried out once a week and subsequent sessions were performed every two weeks. Cognitive stimulation exercises were selected on the basis of the person with dementia's cognitive status profile (Matsuda and Nakatani, 2004). These exercises focused on three different cognitive activities: communication, story learning and word fluency. This study showed a decrease in the MMSE score in the control group that received only pharmacological treatment, but no change in the combined treatment group. The results suggest the possibility that pharmacological treatment plus cognitive stimulation slowed the rate of cognitive decline more than the administration of drug alone.

In a recent study, the same authors compared the cognitive performance of 31 AD persons treated with 7 weeks of 30 minutes CST sessions plus cholinesterase inhibitor therapy to 18 AD persons treated with pharmacological treatment alone. CST followed the same procedure described above. In this study the authors assessed the cognitive changes using Hasegawa's Dementia Scale-Revised (HDS-R) showing that, exclusively in the combined treatment group, a significant cognitive improvement was present (Matsuda et al., 2010). A detailed neuropsychological evaluation could have highlighted further differences between the two experimental groups.

Recently, Giordano and co-workers (2010) compared the efficacy of pharmacological treatment plus an intensive training program including ROT and physical reactivation sessions, with active participation of the caregiver, and pharmacological treatment alone in AD. For this purpose, 100 persons with probable mild to moderate AD were enrolled. All persons with dementia initiated treatment with cholinesterase inhibitors and were allocated to different types of treatment; 62 of them regularly attended daily 45-min class meetings of ROT together with physical reactivation training with the caregiver. Thirty-eight persons with dementia received only cholinesterase inhibitors therapy. All persons with dementia were tested for cognitive and functional abilities at baseline, at the end of the training program (3 weeks) and after 2 months of follow-up. The results showed that persons with dementia that underwent combined treatment with pharmacological therapy plus an intensive program of ROT and physical reactivation sessions performed better than persons with dementia receiving the drug alone, in whom no significant changes in cognition were observed. In particular, persons with dementia showed a significant improvement in MMSE and ADAS-Cog after combined training. Moreover, in these persons with dementia, MMSE improvement was maintained 2 months after the end of the treatment. Conversely, there were no significant changes in the control group that received only cholinesterase inhibitors therapy. These findings suggest that the association of non-pharmacologic and pharmacologic programs is useful for persons with dementia with mild to moderate AD. An additional group of persons with dementia treated with the ROT treatment alone would be useful in order to have completely disentangle the benefits of the combined treatment due to ROT treatment from those provided by the cholinesterase inhibitors therapy.

Conclusion

In conclusion, these studies have suggested that non-pharmacological intervention enhances the effect of cholinesterase inhibitor treatment. Generally, all the studies reported in this review have compared the combined treatment with pharmacological intervention alone. Some of these have included additional control groups (i.e. cognitive treatment alone) in order to verify the improvements induced by the specific cognitive training used, strengthening their results.

Cognitive stimulation, cognitive rehabilitation and cognitive exercise are commonly used nonspecific terms that encompass disparate interventions based on different theoretical constructs. From this point comes a considerable confusion in the terminology used in the researches that combined cognitive intervention and pharmacological treatment. The principal limitation of a critical review is the use of the label of "cognitive approach" for different forms of cognitive intervention. As a further limitation, a crucial issue in non-pharmacological rehabilitation is the long-term duration of the induced effects, although, given the demanding nature of these studies, only a few studies considered more than one follow-up strategy.

An additional factor for consideration is the heterogeneity of methodological conditions used (blindness, control treatment conditions, treatment duration, assessment). Finally, most of the studies that have investigated the additive effects of combined treatment in AD involved relatively small numbers of persons with dementia in each treatment condition and this could represent a limitation.

A recent review (Olazaran et al., 2010) concluded that non-pharmacological therapies can make contributions to the improvement and provision of care for people with AD and their caregivers. The authors highlighted that non-pharmacological and pharmacological therapies should be considered as complementary approaches rather than alternative protocols. Further studies, taking into account the previously highlighted limitations, should clarify the potential role of the combined cognitive-pharmacological treatment in persons with dementia care. In the meantime, the findings of the studies reviewed in this paper suggest that cognitive rehabilitation should be an essential part of dementia treatment, along with anti-dementia drugs.

References

Bottino, C. M., Carvalho, I. A., Alvarez, A. M., Avila, R., Zukauskas, P. R., Bustamante, S. E., Andrade, F. C., Hototian, S. R., Saffi, F., and Camargo, C. H. (2005). Cognitive rehabilitation combined with drug treatment in Alzheimer's disease patients: a pilot study. *Clin Rehabil, 19*(8), 861-869.

Buschert, V., Bokde, A. L., and Hampel, H. (2010). Cognitive intervention in Alzheimer disease. *Nat Rev Neurol, 6*(9), 508-517.

Chapman, S. B., Weiner, M. F., Rackley, A., Hynan, L. S., and Zientz, J. (2004). Effects of cognitive-communication stimulation for Alzheimer's disease patients treated with donepezil. *J Speech Lang Hear Res, 47*(5), 1149-1163.

Cotelli, M., Calabria, M., and Zanetti, O. (2006). Cognitive rehabilitation in Alzheimer's Disease. *Aging Clin Exp Res, 18*(2), 141-143.

Folstein, M. F., Folstein, S. E., and McHugh, P. R. (1975). "Mini-mental state". A practical method for grading the cognitive state of patients for the clinician. *J Psychiatr Res, 12*(3), 189-198.

Giordano, M., Dominguez, L. J., Vitrano, T., Curatolo, M., Ferlisi, A., Di Prima, A., Belvedere, M., and Barbagallo, M. (2010). Combination of intensive cognitive rehabilitation and donepezil therapy in Alzheimer's disease (AD). *Arch Gerontol Geriatr, 51*(3), 245-249.

Matsuda, O. (2007). Cognitive stimulation therapy for Alzheimer's disease: the effect of cognitive stimulation therapy on the progression of mild Alzheimer's disease in patients treated with donepezil. *Int Psychogeriatr, 19*(2), 241-252.

Matsuda, O., and Nakatani, M. (2004). *Manual for Japanese version of the Neurobehavioral Cognitive Status Examination (COGNISTAT)*. Tokyo: World Planning.

Matsuda, O., Shido, E., Hashikai, A., Shibuya, H., Kouno, M., Hara, C., and Saito, M. (2010). Short-term effect of combined drug therapy and cognitive stimulation therapy on the cognitive function of Alzheimer's disease. *Psychogeriatrics, 10*(4), 167-172.

National Institute for Health and Clinical Excellence (2006). *Dementia. Supporting people with dementia and their carers in health and social care [CG42]*. London: National Institute for Health.

Olazaran, J., Reisberg, B., Clare, L., Cruz, I., Pena-Casanova, J., Del Ser, T., Woods, B., Beck, C., Auer, S., Lai, C., Spector, A., Fazio, S., Bond, J., Kivipelto, M., Brodaty, H., Rojo, J. M., Collins, H., Teri, L., Mittelman, M., Orrell, M., Feldman, H. H., and Muniz, R. (2010). Nonpharmacological therapies in Alzheimer's disease: a systematic review of efficacy. *Dement Geriatr Cogn Disord, 30*(2), 161-178.

Onder, G., Zanetti, O., Giacobini, E., Frisoni, G. B., Bartorelli, L., Carbone, G., Lambertucci, P., Silveri, M. C., and Bernabei, R. (2005). Reality orientation therapy combined with cholinesterase inhibitors in Alzheimer's disease: randomised controlled trial. *Br J Psychiatry, 187*, 450-455.

Requena, C., Lopez Ibor, M. I., Maestu, F., Campo, P., Lopez Ibor, J. J., and Ortiz, T. (2004). Effects of cholinergic drugs and cognitive training on dementia. *Dement Geriatr Cogn Disord, 18*(1), 50-54.

Requena, C., Maestu, F., Campo, P., Fernandez, A., and Ortiz, T. (2006). Effects of cholinergic drugs and cognitive training on dementia: 2-year follow-up. *Dement Geriatr Cogn Disord, 22*(4), 339-345.

Rosen, W. G., Mohs, R. C., and Davis, K. L. (1984). A new rating scale for Alzheimer's disease. *Am J Psychiatry, 141*(11), 1356-1364.

Spector, A., Orrell, M., Davies, S., and Woods, B. (2004). Reality Orientation for dementia (Cochrane Review). In *The Cochrane Library, Issue 4*. Chichester, UK: John Wiley and Sons, Ltd.

Tarraga, L., Boada, M., Modinos, G., Espinosa, A., Diego, S., Morera, A., Guitart, M., Balcells, J., Lopez, O. L., and Becker, J. T. (2006). A randomised pilot study to assess the efficacy of an interactive, multimedia tool of cognitive stimulation in Alzheimer's disease. *J Neurol Neurosurg Psychiatry, 77*(10), 1116-1121.

In: Non-Pharmacological Therapies .. . ISBN: 978-1-63321-860-4
Editor: Elisabetta Farina

Chapter 7

Cognitive Rehabilitation in Mild Cognitive Impairment: A Pilot Study

Elena Farini, Paola Frasson, Giada Caramatti, Eleonora Catricalà, Jubin Abutalebi, Alessandra Marcone and Stefano F. Cappa
Università Vita-Salute San Raffaele, Department of Neuroscience,
Scientific Institute H S. Raffaele – Milan. Italy

Abstract

Introduction. There is some evidence that cognitive rehabilitation can delay cognitive and functional decline in healthy older adults and person living with Alzheimer's disease (AD). Persons living with mild cognitive impairment (MCI) usually retain a wide range of cognitive capacities, and may thus represent an ideal target for cognitive rehabilitation.

Aim. To investigate the effectiveness of a 8-week cognitive rehabilitation program in persons living with MCI.

Subjects and methods. The study included an experimental group of 10 subjects (5 with Amnestic MCI -a-MCI- and 5 with amnestic multi-domain MCI -amd-MCI) and a control group of 5 comparable subjects (2 with a-MCI and 3 with amd-MCI). The experimental and control group were matched for Mini Mental State Examination (MMSE) score, years of education, age, basic activities of daily living (BADL), and instrumental activities of daily living (IADL). The rehabilitation program included a computerized cognitive rehabilitation program, drills with graded levels of difficulty, homework and specific instructions about the use of the strategies in real-life situations.

Results. The study outcome measures were the scores on neuropsychological tests as well as the functional status (IADL, BADL), which were assessed prior to enrolment, at the end of the rehabilitation program and after 2 months. In the experimental group the 2 months follow-up assessment revealed no significant differences in neuropsychological tests, except for a significant improvement in phonemic verbal fluency. In contrast, the controls showed a worsening of performance in semantic and phonemic verbal fluency and in IADL at the time of the third evaluation, two months after the end of treatment. One of the trained MCI and 3 out of 5 control subjects progressed to AD during the period of the study.

Conclusion. The results of this pilot study suggest that a comprehensive cognitive rehabilitation program may have beneficial effects on cognitive function and functional status in both a-MCI and amd-MCI subjects.

Keywords: Cognitive rehabilitation, Mild Cognitive Impairment (MCI), Alzheimer's disease (AD)

Introduction

Mild Cognitive Impairment (MCI) is associated with a high risk of progression to dementia and, in particular, to Alzheimer's disease (AD). It is estimated that between 20 to 50% of persons living with MCI progress to AD over a period of 2-3 years [1,2]. At the moment, no effective pharmacological treatment is available to stop or delay this progression. Acetylcholinesterase inhibitors (AChEI) have not been shown to be effective in a large clinical trial [3,4]. There is some evidence that cognitive training and rehabilitation can delay cognitive and functional decline in healthy older adults and even in person with dementia [5]. While the results of the Cochrane review are inconclusive [4], a large effect size has been reported in many studies [6,7].

This finding has important consequences for its potential application to MCI. Indeed, persons fulfilling the criteria for MCI retain a large range of cognitive capacities, and may thus represent an ideal target for cognitive training and rehabilitation. In a recent systematic review [7] the authors considered 15 papers in which the efficacy of cognitive intervention programs has been tested in persons with amnestic MCI (a-MCI). The data showed statistically significant improvements at the end of training in 44% objective measures of memory and in 49% of subjective measures of memory, quality of life and mood. The conclusions of this review recommends that we need studies in randomised trials of large samples of subjects employing standardized and validated objective (standardized neuropsychological tests) and subjective (quality of life, mood and functional impact scales) measures of efficacy in different domains (cognition, everyday life and affective symptoms). New trials should also include a follow-up to assess the long-term persistence of rehabilitation effects. Noteworthy, the type of sessions (group or individual) does not seem to influence the efficacy. Recommendations are also provided regarding the neuropsychological battery that should be employed, i.e., batteries including sensitive and specific assessments of memory and executive functions. A further recent review [6] targeting memory rehabilitation in MCI individuals, analysed, using a priori criteria, a total of 226 studies, 10 of which were included in the final analysis. The conclusions were limited, due to the poor methodological quality of many studies, and suggested that persons with MCI can learn specific information relevant to the individual and, probably, compensatory strategies for memory deficits. However, only limited evidence is available indicating that memory training can generalize and the findings regarding the impact on everyday life are contradictory.

At the practical level, programs with a number of sessions between 6 and 20 that last less than 12 weeks seem to be a rational choice in terms of cost/effectiveness and of compliance of involved persons. We report here the result of a pilot study investigating the effectiveness of a 8-weeks cognitive rehabilitation program in persons living with MCI as compared to age-matched person with dementia who did not undergo any specific rehabilitation.

Subject and Methods

The participants in the study were selected according to Petersen's most recent criteria [1,2] for a-MCI and amd-MCI. The diagnosis was based on a thorough neurological and neuropsychological assessment. Further, all participants underwent CT scanning to exclude the presence of other brain diseases. All participants reported pathological scores, corrected for age and education, on Rey word list (immediate and delayed recall) in agreement with Carlesimo et al. [16]. All participants had scores above the age- and education corrected cut off for dementia on the MMSE [10]. None of the participants reported a significant impact of the cognitive deficits upon functional independence as evaluated through the use of clinical interviews both with the person with dementia themselves and their relatives. Vascular lesions in the brain and depression were exclusion criteria. All participants were monolingual Italians with normal visual and auditory acuity. None of the participants was under treatment with acetylcholinesterase inhibitors or antidepressant drugs. The experimental group included 10 subjects, 5 with a-MCI and 5 with amd-MCI. The control group included 5 not-trained persons: 2 with a-MCI and 3 with amd-MCI. The subjects in the control group could not participate in the rehabilitation program because they were living far from Milan.

There were six males in the trained MCI group and five males in the non-trained MCI group. At the time of the first assessment the two groups were well-matched for Mini Mental State Examination (MMSE) ($p=0.513$), education ($p=0.594$), age ($p=0.206$) and years post-onset ($p= 0,953$). Clinical and demographic data are reported in Table1.

All subjects were administered a neuropsychological and functional assessment. The neuropsychologist administering the assessment was not involved in cognitive rehabilitation. The neuropsychological battery included: MMSE [10], token test [11,12], phonemic and semantic verbal fluency [13], digit forward [14], digit backward [15], Corsi test [14], Rey word list (immediate and delayed) [16], Rey complex figure (immediate and delayed) [17], Raven's progressive matrices [12], attentional matrices [12].

Basic Activities of Daily living (BADL) and Instrumental Activities of Daily living (IADL) were assessed with an informant interview [18,19]. All subjects included in the study were rated as questionable dementia (0.5) on the Clinical Dementia Rating (CDR) [20].

The complete evaluation was carried out for each participant before and after treatment (respectively T0 and T1) and 2 months after the end of treatment (T2). It was not possible to administer the neuropsychological and functional assessment to 3 out of the 10 trained a-MCI subjects at T2, in one cause because the person with dementia was in hospital for an orthopaedic emergency and in two others because they had moved away from Milan.

Data were analysed using SPSS 15.0 software for Windows. We compared the performances obtained by the two groups on each test at the three times of assessment (T0, T1 and T2) separately, using the Mann-Whitney test. A Friedman Test was carried out in order to compare observations at the three different periods (T0, T1 and T2) on 7 trained MCI and on 5 untrained MCI, separately for each test. In order to compare performances obtained at two different periods, e.g. T0 and T1, T1 and T2 and T0 and T2, we used the Wilcoxon test.

Note that, because of the lack of tests scores at T2 for 3 of the 10 trained MCI, only the comparison between T0 and T1 could be performed on 10 trained MCI. The two other comparisons were carried out for only 7 trained MCI.

Table 1. Clinical and demographic characteristics of the groups at T0

	MCI TRAINED Mean (sd)	MCI NOT TRAINED Mean (sd)	p
Age	70,9 (4,84)	75,60 (6,23)	0,206
Education	9,5 (3,17)	9,2 (5,22)	0,594
MMSE (uncorrected score)	24,6 (1,51)	24 (2)	0,513
BADL	6	6	1
IADL	8	8	1

The rehabilitation program lasted 8 weeks. Each rehabilitation session was individual, occurred once a week, and lasted 60 minutes. The individual rehabilitation program consisted of drills with graded levels of difficulty, homework, specific instructions about the use of the strategies in real-life situations, and computerized cognitive training programs from COGPACK [8]. Cogpack consists of 64 programs for testing and training, each with several variants and difficulty levels for visuomotor, comprehension, reaction times, vigilance, memory, language, intellectual and professional skills. Exercises can be varied by random routines and user-edited exercise material. Instructions, timing, type and scope of exercise series, as well as the exercises themselves can be altered. Score reporting is automatic and supplies both completion times for each task and the corresponding scores. The use and results of all these resources was noted daily for the purpose of a constant qualitative appraisal of any and all changes within each participants cognitive profile.

In accordance with the cognitive profile resulting from the initial neuropsychological evaluation, the rehabilitation program aimed at strengthening the defective cognitive areas, optimising residual cognitive potential and creating compensatory strategies. Each rehabilitation session was structured with the aim to stimulate all deficient cognitive areas within the same sitting. The amount of time dedicated to the stimulation of each deficient cognitive area was dependent on the individual's specific cognitive profile.

The first part of each rehabilitation session was dedicated to the orientation of the participant, aiming at the improvement of spatial, temporal and personal awareness. The rehabilitation was based on an explicit verbal learning of information pertaining to dates and places of interest to the individual and to his or her personal or familiar history. To this end, calendars and photographs were employed as external aids.

Once sufficient time, in accordance with the needs of each individual, had been dedicated to orientation training, the sessions continued with the rehabilitation of memory skills. Memory rehabilitation training was based on a series of methods, all aiming to boost mnestic functions and to improve recall. This was achieved by supplying the participant with techniques facilitating the use of residual memory resources with the aim to transfer the acquired abilities into activities of daily living. Some of the cognitive techniques used were: spaced-retrieval (methods based on augmenting recall abilities through learning of information and retrieval of the same material after increasing periods of time), category cue (methods based on the categorical organization of information), visual imagery (methods based on the association of visual images to verbal material in order to facilitate learning), and methods based on implicit memory. We trained the acquisition and recall of word lists, word pairs, prose material (short stories, books and newspaper articles), as well as of visuo-spatial material. External passive aids [9], such as adaptation of environmental conditions and reality orientation, and external active aids, such as datebooks, timers, calendars, shopping and 'to do' lists were also utilized, as well as memory subprograms from COGPACK [8], such as word lists, images and labels, patterns, signs, addresses, routes, and lively scenes.

Alternating with memory rehabilitation tasks within the same session, the rehabilitation of attentional resources included several tasks. Focal and/or selective attention required visual or acoustic target identification among a series of verbal or non-verbal stimuli, presented on paper or on a computer screen (Vigilance sub-programs from COGPACK), which could vary according to number or complexity. The same tasks could be repeated with the introduction of interference or interruptions.

For the amd-MCI participant group, additional rehabilitation areas were included into each rehabilitation session in accordance with each participant's specific cognitive profile. These included training of language and of logical and visuo-spatial abilities.

Language training involved the use of exercises for production and comprehension. For verbal production, the individual was asked to name visual and verbal stimuli, using the cueing technique, and to retrieve lexical items on the basis of semantic and phonemic cues. Comprehension abilities were trained with simple and complex questions.

Training of logical and abstraction abilities was based on the use of tasks of categorization, problem solving, calculation, association, analogy, metaphor and proverb comprehension.

Training of visuo-spatial abilities included visual exploration tasks and praxic-constructive tasks (puzzles, copy and completion of figures, labyrinths, etc.).

As a general rule, all deficient cognitive areas were stimulated within each rehabilitation session, but the time allotted to each cognitive function was dependent on the individual's specific cognitive profile. However, because the participant population consists of individuals living with a-MCI, a larger portion of time was dedicated to memory tasks and, to a lesser degree, to attentional resources, compared to the remaining cognitive areas.

Results

During the period of the study, 3 out of the 5 persons in the control group progressed to a diagnosis of probable AD, while only one of the trained MCI progressed to AD.

Comparisons of cognitive and functional status between trained MCI group and controls at each of the tree time intervals (T0, T1, T2) for each test are shown in Table 2.

At T0, no significant differences were found between the two groups for any neuropsychological test, with the exception of immediate Rey list (p=0,038), with a better performance for the trained group. At T1, trained MCI had higher scores than controls on the IADL (p=0,013), at T2 on IADL (p=0,009), token test (p=0,048) and phonemic fluency (p=0,018).

Considering the longitudinal profile (T0, T1 and T3) of the two groups separately, we observed a significant improvement in the trained MCI group on phonemic fluency (p=0,05). In contrast, a significant decline was evident in the control group on IADL (p=0,014) and semantic fluency (p=0,015). Phonemic fluency approached significance (p=0,074). In order to investigate at which assessment the differences became significant, we compared the scores obtained at T0 and T1, T0 and T2 and T1 and T2, for each group separately. Comparisons between T0 and T1 showed no significant difference in the trained group, while the control group obtained a worse performance on semantic fluency (p=0,043). The difference in IADL (p=0,068) approached significance. Considering the T1 and T2 periods, trained MCI showed a trend towards a better performance in T2 than T1 on phonemic fluency (p=0,062). Finally, the performance at T2 was not different from that of T0 on all tests in trained MCI. In contrast, the control group showed a lower score at T2 than T0 on IADL (p=0,042), semantic (p=0,043) and phonemic fluency (p=0,043).

Finally, there were no differences in either demographic variables (age, education) or pre-training neuropsychological measures between those persons who converted from MCI to dementia (1 out of the experimental group and 3 out of the control group) and those who did not convert.

Conclusion

In the present study, we provide preliminary evidence about the cognitive and functional impact of a two months program of weekly cognitive rehabilitation in persons living with MCI, compared with a non-trained, matched MCI control group.

Overall, a stabilization of cognitive abilities and functional status between baseline and follow-up was observed in the trained group. In contrast, non trained MCI persons showed not only a decline in test performances, but also a significant worsening in instrumental activities of daily living. In fact, three subjects from the control group progressed to a clinical diagnosis of probable AD at follow-up, while only one of the trained MCI showed the same progression.

Participants who converted from MCI to AD did not differ from those not converted in AD (8 participants) in either demographic variables (age, education) or in the pre-training neuropsychological measures. The non-trained MCI who converted into AD group were all a-mdMCI. In fact, the multiple domain type of MCI has a less favourable prognosis then amnestic type and may represent a more advanced prodromal stage of dementia [21,22].

Given that the functional status and the neuropsychological profile in treated and non treated persons was similar at baseline, we can conclude that our results are in agreement with others studies that demonstrated the efficacy of cognitive interventions in persons with MCI on various cognitive performances [23,24,25,26].

For example, Belleville et al. [23] focused on teaching episodic memory strategies, comparing the performance of trained MCI persons with an untrained control group. A significant pre-post intervention improvement was observed in delayed list recall and face-name association. Talassi et al. [26] reported the effectiveness of neuropsychological rehabilitation on cognitive and behavioural symptoms and functional status in a group of person living with MCI and mild dementia. Their results demonstrated that a systematic rehabilitation program results in an improvement in Rey figure copy and recall, and in a significant reduction of depression and anxiety symptoms. Rozzini et al. [25] reported a one year longitudinal study of neuropsychological training in 59 person living with MCI treated with cholinesterase inhibitors.

Table 2. Comparison of cognitive and functional status in trained and not trained MCI group at the tree time intervals (T0, T1, T2); p values based on Friedman non parametric test; DS= Digit Span; sd = standard deviation; NS= not significant

Parameters	EXPERIMENTAL GROUP Mean (sd)				CONTROL GROUP Mean (sd)			
	At time T0	At time T1	At time T2	p	At time T0	At time T1	At time T2	p
Cognitive functions								
MMSE score	24,6 (1,51)	23,60 (2,46)	23,57 (4,54)	NS	24 (2)	23,2 (2,78)	22,4 (2,88)	NS
Token Test	31,50 (2,14)	30,69 (2,02)	31 (4,87)	NS	32 (2,45)	27,8 (4,55)	26,7 (2,11)	0,076
Phonemic verbal fluency	24,7 (10,32)	23,4 (11,2)	29,57 (10,94)	0,05	22,6 (8,47)	17,2 (7,19)	13 (9,22)	0,074
Semantic verbal fluency	25,5 (6,77)	24,4 (7,99)	23,29 (7,59)	NS	30 (6,82)	21 (6,40)	18 (11,14)	0,015
DS forward	5,1 (0,57)	5,1 (0,74)	5,14 (0,69)	NS	5,2 (0,84)	5 (0,7)	4,8 (0,84)	NS
DS backward	3,78 (0,68)	3,7 (0,48)	3,43 (0,79)	NS	3,2 (0,45)	3,2 (0,84)	2,8 (0,84)	NS
Corsi Test	4,6 (0,84)	4,4 (0,52)	4,57 (0,53)	NS	4,2 (0,45)	4,2 (0,84)	3,8 (1,1)	NS
Rey List immediate recall	24,67 (8,07)	25,25 (6,45)	24,33 (11,46)	NS	13 (5,29)	15,4 (6,8)	18 (5,34)	NS
Rey List delayed recall	0,5 (0,84)	0,38 (0,74)	0,33 (0,52)	NS	1 (2)	0	0,4 (0,89)	NS
Figure Rey Copy	31,85 (2,54)	30,8 (4,32)	31,93 (3,79)	NS	32,6 (2,51)	23,9 (14,51)	25 (8,92)	NS
Figure Rey Recall	7,15 (4,39)	6,40 (5,64)	5,14 (4,46)	NS	8,7 (7,4)	7,6 (7,85)	5,3 (5,7)	NS
Raven Test	25,5 (4,17)	23,5 (5,62)	23,14 (7,01)	NS	24 (2,55)	18,6 (6,84)	19,6 (8,26)	NS
Attentive Matrices	45,4 (6,08)	42,6 (6,07)	45,14 (8,36)	NS	44 (4,3)	39,2 (15,48)	36 (12,41)	NS
Functional Status								
BADL	6	6	6	NS	6	5,8 (0,45)	5,6 (0,89)	NS
IADL	8	8	7,5 (1,23)	NS	8	5,4 (2,41)	4,4 (1,82)	0,014

Subjects treated with cognitive training and cholinesterase inhibitors showed significant improvements in memory, abstract reasoning and depressive symptoms, while no improvement was found in the controls.

The lack of improvement in the memory measures found in our study may be attributed to a floor effect present in both groups at T0. However, a trend towards a worse performance at T2 than T1 was observed in not-trained MCI on Rey figure recall. The only significant improvement was found for phonemic fluency. In contrast, both phonemic and semantic fluency declined in the controls. These data corroborate other findings [24] showing a positive effect of a three months computer-based cognitive rehabilitation on the area of verbal production, in particular on phonemic fluency, in 10 person with AD, and on the area of memory in 10 persons with MCI. These data seem to indicate that the same individualized rehabilitative intervention could have different effects according to the participant's diagnosis.

One limitation of the study is the lack of a true randomization (the controls were not offered the training because of their inability to attend the program). Even more important is the small sample size, which does not allow a generalization of the present results to the MCI population. Nevertheless, when considered together with the other published studies, the present findings support the need to further investigate the possible usefulness of tailored cognitive interventions in MCI.

References

[1] Petersen, R.C.; Smith, G.E.; Waring, S.C.; Ivnik, R.J.; Tangalos, E.G. and Kokmen, E. (1999). Mild cognitive impairment: clinical characterization and outcome. *Archives of Neurology, 56,* 303–308.

[2] Petersen, R.C.; Doody, R.; Kurz, A.; Mohs, R.C.; Morris, J.C.; Rabins, P.V.; Ritchie, K.; Rossor, M.; Thal, L. and Winblad, B. (2001). Current concepts in MCI. *Archives of Neurology, 58,* 1985-1992.

[3] Raschetti, R.; Albanese, E.; Vanacore, N.; Maggini, M. (2007). Cholinesterase inhibitors in MCI: a systematic review of randomized trials. *PLoS Medicine*, 4, e338.

[4] Birks, J. and Flicker, R. (2006). Donepezil in mild cognitive impairment. *Cochrane Database systematic reviews. 19;3*:CD006104.

[5] Sitzer, D.I.; Twamley, E.W. and Jeste, D.V. (2006). Cognitive training in Alzheimer's Disease: a meta-analysis of the literature. *Acta Psychiatrica Scandinavica, 114,* 75-90.

[6] Stott, J. and Spector, A. (2010). A review of effectiveness of memory interventions in mild cognitive impairment (MCI). *International Psychogeriatrics, 15,* 1-13.

[7] Jean, L.; Bergeron, M.E.; Thivierge, S. and Simard, M. (2010). Cognitive intervention programs for individuals with mild cognitive impairment: systematic review of the literature. *American Journal of Geriatric Psychiatry, 18(4),* 281-296.

[8] Marker, K. (2003). *COGPACK Manual Version 5.9*. Ladenburg (Germany): Marker Software.

[9] Mazzucchi, A. (2006). *La riabilitazione neuropsicologica: Premesse teoriche e applicazioni cliniche (2)*. Milan, Italy: Masson Elsevier.

[10] Folstein, M.F.; Folstein, S.E. and McHugh, P.R. (1975). Mini-Mental State: a practical method for grading the cognitive state of patients for the clinician. Journal of psychiatric research, 12 (3), 189–198.

[11] De Renzi, E. and Vignolo, L.A. (1962). The Token Test: a sensitive test to detect receptive disturbances in Aphasia. *Brain, 85,* 665-78.

[12] Spinnler, H. and Tognoni, G. (1987). Taratura e standardizzazione italiana di test neuropsicologici. *Italian journal of neurological sciences, 6.8*, 7-120.

[13] Novelli, G.; Laiacona, M.; Papagno, C.; Vallar, G.; Capitani, E. and Cappa, S.F. (1986). Tre test clinici di memoria verbale a lungo termine. Taratura su soggetti normali. *Archivio di Psicologia Neurologia Psichiatria, 47*, 278-296.

[14] Orsini, A.; Grossi, D.; Capitani, E.; Laiacona, M.; Papagno, C. and Vallar, G. (1987). Verbal and spatial immediate memory span. Normative data from 1355 adults and 1112 children. *Italian Journal of Neurological Sciences, 8,* 539-548.

[15] Mondini, S.; Mapelli, D.; Vestri, A. and Bisiacchi, P. S. (2003). *Esame neuropsicologico breve* [Short neuropsychological evaluation]. Milan, Italy: Raffaello Cortina Editore.

[16] Carlesimo, G.A.; Caltagirone, C. and Gainotti, G. (1996). Mental Deterioration Battery: normative data, diagnostic reliability and qualitative analyses of cognitive impairment. *European Neurology*, 36, 378-384.

[17] Caffarra, P.; Vezzadini, G.; Dieci, F.; Zonato, F. and Venneri A. (2002). Rey-Osterrieth Complex Figure: normative values in an Italian population sample. *Neurological Sciences*, 22, 443-447.

[18] Katz, S.; Ford, A.B.; Moskowitz, R.W.; Jackson, B.A. and Jaffe, M.W. (1963). Studies of illness in the aged. The Index of ADL: a standardized measure of biological and psychosocial function. *JAMA, 185(12)*, 914-919.

[19] Lawton, M.P. and Brody, E.M. (1969). Assessment of older people: Self-maintaining and instrumental activities of daily living. *The Gerontologist*, *9*(3), 179-186.

[20] Morris, J.C. (1993). The Clinical Dementia Rating (CDR): Current version and scoring rules. *Neurology, 43,* 2412-2414.

[21] Alexopoulos, P. ; Grimmer, T. ; Pernaczky, R. (2006). Progression to dementia in clinical subtypes of mild cognitive impairmentDement Geriatr Cogn Disord 22:27-34.

[22] Yaffe, K.; Petersen, M.C.; Landquist, K.; (2006) Subtype of mild cognitive impairment and progression to dementia and death Dement Geriatr Cogn Disord 22:312-319.

[23] Belleville, S.; Gilbert, B.; Fontaine, F.; Gagnon, L.; Menard, E. and Gauthier, S. (2006). Improvement of episodic memory in persons with mild cognitive impairment an healthy older adults: evidence from a cognitive intervention program. *Dementia and Geriatric Cognitive Disorders, 22*,486-499.

[24] Cipriani, G.; Bianchetti, A and Trabucchi, M. (2006). Outcomes of a computer-based cognitive rehabilitation program on Alzheimer's disease patients compared with those on patients affected by mild cognitive impairment. *Archives of Gerontology and Geriatrics, 43,* 327–335.

[25] Rozzini, L.; Costardi, D.; Vicini Chilovi, B.; Franzoni, S.; Trabucchi, M. and Padovani, A. (2007). Efficacy of cognitive rehabilitation in patients with mild cognitive impairment treated with cholinesterase inhibitors. *International Journal of Geriatric Psychiatry, 22*, 356-360.

[26] Talassi, E.; Guerreschi, M.; Feriani, M.; Fedi, V.; Bianchetti, A. and Trabucchi, M.(2007). Effectiveness of a cognitive rehabilitation program in mild dementia (MD) and Mild Cognitive Impairment (MCI): a case control study. *Archives of Gerontology and Geriatrics - Supplement, 1,* 391-399.

In: Non-Pharmacological Therapies ...
Editor: Elisabetta Farina
ISBN: 978-1-63321-860-4

Chapter 8

From Smartphone to External Semantic Memory Device: The Use of New Technologies to Compensate for Semantic Deficits

Sonia Routhier[1*], Joël Macoir[1], Hélène Imbeault[2], Séverine Jacques[1], Hélène Pigot[3], Sylvain Giroux[3], Albert Cau[3] and Nathalie Bier[4]

[1]Centre de recherche de l'Institut Universitaire en Santé Mentale de Québec, Université Laval, Canada
[2]Centre de recherche sur le vieillissement, Canada
Centre de santé et services sociaux–Institut universitaire de gériatrie de Sherbrooke
[3]Laboratoire DOMUS, Université de Sherbrooke, Canada
[4]Centre de recherche, Institut universitaire de gériatrie de Montréal, Université de Montréal, Canada

Abstract

Background: Semantic dementia (SD) is a neurodegenerative disorder characterized by a progressive loss of semantic memory. The components of SD include impaired word comprehension, anomia and difficulties retrieving people's names. To date, most interventions aimed at improving language-based performances (e.g., naming) and often led to modest results. However, people living with SD could benefit from an ecological intervention focusing on compensation for their needs in activities of daily living (ADL). The use of new technologies is an interesting way to achieve such a compensatory approach for ADL in SD.

Aims: The aim of this case study was to investigate the effectiveness of an ecological compensatory and technological intervention in SD rehabilitation. More specifically, the

* Sonia Routhier, Centre de recherche de l'Institut Universitaire en Santé Mentale de Québec , 2601, de la Canardière, Québec, Québec, Canada G1J 2G3 E-mail: sonia.routhier.1@ulaval.ca

goals were to help a person suffering from SD via the use of a smartphone (1) to retrieve people's names, and (2) to find semantic information essential to comprehension and naming.

Methods: ND is a 51 year-old man who has suffered from SD for 5 years. At baseline, daily self-report measures were used to document the number of times he could not retrieve a person's name and the number of times he used a paper notebook with personal clues to retrieve a name. The number of times he used a paper dictionary to find semantic information essential to comprehension and naming was also measured. The paper notebook and paper dictionary were two self-developed compensatory strategies. The intervention consisted of introducing a smartphone equipped with a new application called ARCUS and with Internet access. ARCUS is a virtual name directory allowing searching for names using personal cues. Daily self-report measures were taken for 2 months after the introduction of the device to measure concurrent use of the smartphone and the previous self-developed compensatory strategies.

Results: A sharp increase in the general tendency to compensate for name-finding difficulties was noted after the introduction of the smartphone. A large general preference for the smartphone over the paper notebook and paper dictionary was also found. The effectiveness of the smartphone and its ease of use were also very satisfactory.

Conclusion: New technologies such as smartphones can be an efficient compensatory intervention in SD. Focusing on the person's needs, the smartphone allowed ND to efficiently compensate for his difficulties in retrieving people's names and to find semantic information essential to word comprehension and naming. New technologies may have a central role to play in SD rehabilitation by providing a fast, efficient, mobile, accessible, ecological and non-stigmatizing way to compensate for deficits.

Keywords: Semantic dementia, management, intervention, smartphone, technologies, language

Introduction

Semantic dementia (SD), one variant of frontotemporal dementia, is a neurodegenerative disorder associated with focal anterior temporal lobe atrophy and characterized by a progressive loss of semantic memory (Gorno-Tempini et al., 2011; Neary et al., 1998). The principal complaint usually concerns language difficulties, particularly in understanding and finding words (Hodges, Patterson, Oxbury, and Funnel, 1992). The main diagnosis components of SD are impaired word comprehension, anomia, prosopagnosia (inability to recognize faces) and associative agnosia (inability to recognize objects) (Gorno-Tempini et al., 2011; Neary et al., 1998; Burrell and Hodges, 2010). Clinical observations show that people living with SD also report difficulties retrieving people's names (proper name anomia). Comprehension deficits are not always apparent in spontaneous speech or conversation because production is fluent and contextual information aids comprehension. However, people living with SD show substantial difficulties in all tasks requiring the activation of semantic information (e.g., word definition, picture naming, semantic questionnaires, word comprehension) (Breedin, Saffran, and Coslett, 1994; Hodges and Graham, 1998; Hodges, Patterson, and Tyler, 1994; Hodges, Graham, and Patterson, 1995; Hodges, Patterson et al., 1992; Snowden, Griffiths, and Neary, 1994). Other cognitive abilities like executive functions, episodic memory, time orientation and space orientation, as well as perceptual and praxis skills are usually preserved in SD (Neary et al., 1998). However, cognitive functions and praxis requiring semantic knowledge are also affected. For example, people living with SD show impairment in using objects for which they present difficulties activating semantic knowledge (Bozeat, Lambon Ralph, Patterson, and Hodges, 2002; Hamanaka et al., 1996; Hodges et al., 2000).

The clinical symptoms of SD affect activities of daily living (ADL) but, to date, these consequences are not well documented. People living with SD may show deficits with complex and language-based activities like using a telephone, cooking, managing their money or grocery shopping (Bier and Macoir, 2010; Mioshi et al., 2007; Moishi and Hodges, 2009). Significant changes in everyday behaviours such as neglecting hygiene or being more selective in the choice of food have also been reported (Snowden et al., 2001; Shinagawa, Ikeda, Fukuhara, and Tanabe, 2006; Kashibayashi et al., 2010).

To date, interventions in SD mainly aimed at improving language-based performance (e.g., Croot, Nikels, Laurence, and Manning, 2009) or focused on the use of objects (Bozeat, Patterson, and Hodges, 2004; Robinson, Druks, Hodges, and Garrard, 2009). Even if language enhancement in SD is possible, most studies have demonstrated that improvements are often modest, with poor maintenance after the end of treatment, no generalization to untreated items and frequent reliance on specific temporo-spatial contexts (Funnell, 1995; Graham, Patterson, Pratt, and Hodges, 1999, 2001; Jokel, Rochon, and Leonard, 2002, 2006; Snowden and Neary, 2002; Frattali et al., 2004; Henry, Besson, and Rapcsak, 2008; Bier et al., 2009). For example, in a person living with SD Funnell (1995) noted the maintenance of naming improvement (6/6) 1 week after the therapy ended, followed 2 (5/6) and 8 (3/6) months later by a progressive decrease. This pattern of decline was also reported in most studies (Bier et al., 2009; Frattali, 2004; Graham et al., 1999, 2001; Jokel et al., 2002, 2006; Snowden and Neary, 2002). However, Jokel et al. (2007, 2010) reported the case of CS, a person living with SD, for whom therapeutic gains lasted and generalized to a new context, using a computer-based errorless approach. Heredia et al. (2009) reported the same relearning pattern in the case of CUB using a conventional naming therapy ("look and say" method). Nevertheless, as reported by Henry et al. (2008) and Dewar et al. (2009), the relearned information in cases of progressive language impairment may differ qualitatively from the rich original semantic representations present before the onset of SD.

Because of the cognitive characteristics of the disease and the difficulties encountered in ADL, people living with SD could benefit from an ecological intervention that focuses on their specific needs and deficits in everyday living. In SD, few treatment studies have been conducted with an ecological or compensatory approach. As an exception, Bier, Macoir, and Joubert (2011) showed that EC, a woman with SD, could relearn how to cook two recipes and reintegrate them in her day-to-day life. The therapy used with EC consisted of preparing a recipe and encouraging her to cook as often as possible. The therapy included a target and control recipes, that were practised, and two neutral, non-practised recipes. With this approach, EC significantly increased the amount of relevant information she could provide about food items included in the recipes practised, but could not provide such information for the ingredients of the neutral recipes. She also significantly increased the number of meals spontaneously cooked between therapy sessions. This ecological approach appeared to be effective with this person. Its relevance for SD, therefore, warrants further study.

Using new technologies is another approach that can be helpful in managing cognitive impairments in degenerative disorders. For example, cellphones have been useful in compensating for memory deficits in Alzheimer's disease (Lekeu, Wojtasik, Van der Linden, and Salmon, 2002; Quittre, Adam, Olivier, and Salmon, 2009; Imbeault et al., 2011), with the further advantage of being non-stigmatizing. In 2009, Svoboda and Richards used a smartphone with RR, a person suffering from anterograde amnesia and space disorientation following brain surgery. The authors reported successful results for objective and qualitative measures of memory functioning. Generalization was also seen across different real-life memory-demanding circumstances for which RR did not receive any training. This example shows the auspicious effect new technologies could have in an ecological intervention approach. The use of such external aids to facilitate the autonomy of people living with SD in their day-to-day lives has not yet been studied.

The aim of the present study was thus to investigate the effectiveness of an ecological, compensatory intervention in SD rehabilitation employing new technologies to compensate for the negative impact of semantic memory deficits on ADL. More specifically, this case study aimed at helping an individual suffering from SD, via the use of a smartphone, to retrieve the names of people met at work (Study 1) and to find semantic information essential to comprehension and naming (Study 2).

Methods

Case Description

ND is a 51 year-old man, native speaker of French, right-handed, with a 14 years of education. He had managed a seniors' home for about 20 years. He then worked as a recreation therapist in a seniors' home since 2009. ND presented to us in September 2009 with a 2-year history of cognitive decline. He complained of word-finding problems, impaired comprehension and difficulties in recognizing and naming people. When we saw him, ND lived with his wife in an apartment, continued to work 4 days a week and was still doing the housework, cooking and shopping, as well as managing the household finances. He continued to use his car and ride his bicycle.

Neuropsychological assessment. In September 2009, ND underwent a complete neuropsychological examination. His performance on neuropsychological tests is shown in Table 1.

With respect to memory, ND was well oriented in time and space but reported occasional difficulties in recognizing well-known people. ND's performance on visual episodic memory (DMS-48; Barbeau et al., 2004) was well preserved in immediate and delayed recognition phases but he was impaired on verbal episodic memory subtests (logical memory) of the PENO battery (Joanette et al., 1995). Working memory, measured using forward and backward digit span, was intact. His performance was also within the normal range for tasks exploring motor control. With respect to executive functions, his performance was good for tests exploring mental flexibility (Trail making test; Reitan, 1958), spatial planning (D-Kefs tower test; Delis, Kaplan, and Kramer, 2001), inhibition (Stroop test; Golden, 1978), and rule detection (Brixton spatial anticipation test; Burgess and Shallice, 1997). Visual-perceptual abilities also appeared to be well preserved, except for object decision tasks of the BORB battery (Riddoch and Humphreys, 1993).

With regard to language, speech output was fluent, well-articulated and grammatically correct but presented many signs of word-finding difficulties: miscarried sentences, latencies and occasional semantic paraphasias. ND's performance for the auditory (18/20) lexical decision task was slightly below the normal range (19.86; SD = .38) whilst he performed normally on the written lexical decision task (19/20) (BECLA; Macoir, Gauthier, and Jean, 2005). Word fluency performed with the first letter criterion was poor. Repetition was flawless for words and nonwords. Reading (BECLA) was flawless for nonwords (10/10) and slightly impaired for words (8/10) with production of regularization errors. Written spelling of nonwords was perfectly preserved (10/10) but the results on word writing to dictation was canonical of surface agraphia (16/20). With respect to syntactic comprehension, ND performed flawlessly (13/13) on the written sentence-to-picture matching test (MT86: Nespoulous et al., 1992).

Table 1. ND's performance on neuropsychological tests

	ND	Norm
Episodic/working memory tests		
Digit span forward	8	WNR
Digit span backward	7	WNR
Immediate story retelling subtest (PENO) (24)	7*	12.3 (3.5)
Delayed story retelling subtest (PENO) (24)	5*	9.25 (1.7)
DMS-48 immediate recognition (48)	47	47.52 (.96)
DMS-48 delayed recognition (48)	47	47.52 (.96)
Visual-perceptual tests		
Length match task (BORB) (30)	30	26.9 (1.6)
Object decision – easy subtest (BORB) (32)	27*	30.5 (1.4)
Object decision – hard subtest (BORB) (32)	23*	27.0 (2.2)
Motor control tests		
Copy of the Rey figure (36)	36	32.4 (1.1)
Pantomime imitation subtest (PENO) (35)	33	32.8 (1.8)
Arbitrary gesture imitation subtest (PENO) (35)	35	33.6 (1.1)
Executive functions tests		
Trail Making Test – part A (sec.)	13	31.78 (9.93)
Trail Making Test – part B (sec.)	34	63.76 (14.42)
Stroop Test – word (sec.)	28	42.68 (6.98)
Stroop Test – color (sec.)	55	54.94 (9.43)
Stroop Test - interference (sec.)	104	88.07 (20.47)
D-Kefs Tower – total achievement (scaled score)	15	10 (3)
Brixton Test - scaled score	5	Mod. average
Language tests		
Letter fluency subtest (PENO – letter T)	8*	14.2 (2.3)
Letter fluency subtest (PENO – letter P)	13*	19 (1.7)
Written word and sentence – picture matching (MT-86) (13)	13	12.51 (.91)
Words and nonwords repetition (BECLA) (25)	25	25 (-)
Words and nonwords reading (BECLA) (20)	18*	19.86 (.19)
Word spelling to dictation (BECLA) (20)	16*	19.86 (.38)
Nonword spelling to dictation (BECLA) (10)	10	9.57 (.79)
Semantic memory tests		
Picture naming (TDQ-60) (60)	46*	58.2 (.42)
Pyramids and Palm Trees Test – picture-to-picture substest (52)	37*	49.33 (1.78)
Category fluency subtest (PENO)	24*	48.8 (4.5)

Indicates a score below the norm or outside the normal range; WNR: within the normal range

Finally, ND was impaired on all tasks exploring semantic memory. He encountered serious difficulties in confrontation naming investigated with the TDQ-60 (Macoir, Beaudoin, and Bluteau, 2008). In this task, he produced semantic and visual-semantic paraphasias.

He also showed clear problems with semantic processing on the picture-to-picture matching condition of the Pyramids and Palm Trees Test (Howard and Patterson, 1992). Category fluency was extremely poor.

Neuroimaging. A CT scan done in April 2007 revealed cortical atrophy of the temporal lobes, slightly more prevalent on the left side. A PET scan done in May 2007 showed atrophy of the temporal lobes, most marked anteriorly and more prevalent on the left side.

Summary and diagnosis. Overall, ND presented with deficits on all tests requiring semantic processing and verbal comprehension of words but performed normally on tests exploring visual-perceptual abilities, visual episodic memory, motor control, and executive functions. Along with neuroimagery data, these results were congruent with the clinical characteristics of possible SD (Gorno-Tempini et al., 2011; Neary et al., 1998).

Difficulties in day-to-day life and compensatory strategies. ND presented with substantial difficulties recognizing faces of people he met. His main complaint was his inability to retrieve the names of the residents at the seniors' home. This difficulty was particularly embarrassing because many elders initiated talks with ND, who could not recall their names. To compensate, he used a paper notebook to record residents' names along with personal cues (e.g., hair color, room number) to help him retrieve their names. When a discussion was spontaneously initiated by a resident, ND first used indefinite expressions (e.g., "Hello Sir!") and then unobtrusively looked in his paper notebook for the person's name using the personal clue he remembered. When he knew he would have to talk to a specific person, ND previously looked in his paper notebook to retrieve the name. However, this paper notebook is not very portable and its use is time-consuming. ND also developed other strategies to circumvent his difficulty. For example, he might use a roundabout question or read a resident's name written on a walker. ND also used humour or different excuses (e.g., busy day) when he made errors on proper names, produced semantic paraphasias or could not find a word because of anomia.

ND also presented other difficulties due to semantic impairment. His recreation therapist work required creating and managing various activities (e.g., crossword puzzles, riddles) that included semantic or general culture questions. Because of his semantic impairment, creating these activities necessitated many hours of preparation and planning.

Comprehension difficulties also sometimes appeared in different circumstances when ND failed to retrieve the meaning of a word important to the discussion. At work, he did not have any specific compensatory strategy other than consulting a paper dictionary, when easily accessible, or using a roundabout question to find the meaning of a word. Moreover, his surface dysgraphia made dictionary searching more difficult.

Intervention Description

The specific needs and difficulties of ND were twofold: a) he presented with difficulty retrieving the residents' names of the seniors' home, and b) the semantic deficit made his recreationist work laborious and affected his comprehension and naming in real time. We therefore suggested a specific intervention aimed at compensating for his difficulty in retrieving people's names (Study 1) and compensating for comprehension and naming difficulties (Study 2). What makes this intervention interesting is the use of a smartphone to satisfy both requirements.

In Study 1, to compensate for the difficulty retrieving people's names, the smartphone was equipped with a new application called "ARCUS", a virtual directory of names allowing searching for information using personal cues. The contacts are registered by the subject who uses several optional criteria to specify a new contact, such as age or keywords (description). Searches within contacts are performed with different parameters: name, keyword description, room number, age, birthday, phone number (see Figure 1).

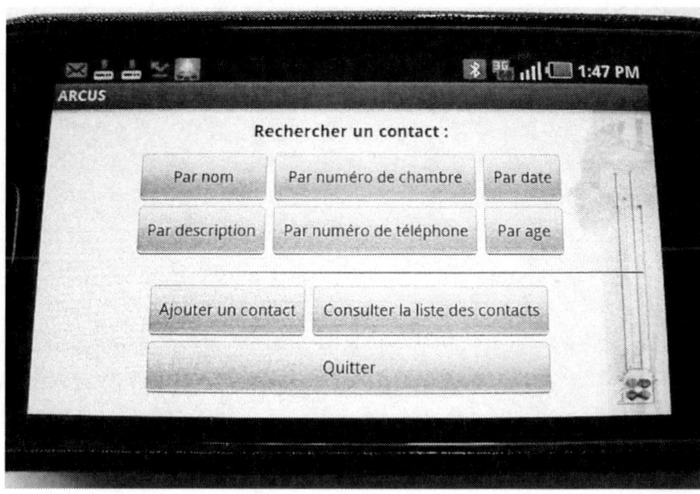

Figure 1. ARCUS home page.

In fact, this application replicates the information contained in ND's paper notebook. However, its aim was to replace the paper notebook with a more convenient and portable external aid.

In Study 2, aimed at compensating for word comprehension and naming difficulties, the smartphone was provided with Internet access in order to search for the meaning of words using search engines or free encyclopaedias (e.g., Google Image, Wikipedia). ND was familiar with the Internet and computer science in general. He sometimes searched the Internet at home on his personal computer to prepare the activities for elders at the seniors' home. However, no Internet access was available for him at work, making it impossible to search for word meanings when necessary.

Goal Summary

The main goal of this experiment was to investigate the effectiveness of an ecological and compensatory intervention in SD rehabilitation, using a smartphone to compensate for the negative impact of semantic memory deficits. In Study 1, the goal was to help ND compensate for the difficulty retrieving people's names at work. More specifically, the goals were a) to measure the changes in the general tendency to compensate when ARCUS was added to the paper notebook as a second possible strategy, b) to compare use of the paper notebook and ARCUS, and c) to measure the effectiveness of ARCUS. In Study 2, aimed at compensating for word comprehension and naming difficulties, the specific goals were a) to measure use of the smartphone to search the Internet, b) to compare use of the Internet and the paper dictionary, and c) to measure the ease of using the smartphone to search the Internet.

Study 1. Inability to Retrieve People's Names: Use of the Paper Notebook and ARCUS

An ABA multiple baseline design (Ottenbacher, 1986; Wilson, 1987) was used. The procedure included (A) baseline measures, (B) intervention consisting of the introduction of a new compensatory strategy and training, and (A) follow-up measures with the compensation strategy.

(A) Baseline. Before the introduction of the smartphone, ND was asked to fill out a daily self-report (one-page table) for two weeks concerning his difficulty retrieving names. More specifically, this self-report provided information about the number of persons whose names ND could not recall during the day and the number of times he used his paper notebook to compensate.

***(B) Intervention*:** Introduction of the smartphone and training. After phase A, the smartphone equipped with ARCUS was given to ND and training was provided. Sohlberg and Mateer (1989) described a structured training method in three steps: acquisition, application and adaptation. Acquisition is a stage of familiarization with the device during which the person learns the different functions of the device. Application is the step in which the person learns in which day-to-day situations he can use the device. Role-plays are often used in this step to allow the subject to experiment in different situations and provide immediate feedback.

Finally, adaptation is the stage at which the person adapts and modifies the learned skills to use them efficiently in real situations. This step is usually performed in community living, supported by the therapist.

This three-step method was chosen to support ND in learning how to use ARCUS and the Internet on his smartphone.

At the beginning, help given to ND was total and he only had to observe the experimenter using ARCUS in order to understand how the application works. Gradually, less help was given until he could use the application on his own (vanishing cues approach). Learning how to use ARCUS (acquisition and application) was done in one intensive 3-hour session. At the end of the session, ND was able to use it on his own, without help.

To optimize use of the smartphone (adaptation), a therapist accompanied ND to work and encouraged him to use the phone. The therapist could also help ND if he had difficulties. The "at work" part of the training lasted 2 weeks, 4 days a week, during normal work hours (~9 a.m. to 4 p.m.).

(A) Follow-up. To obtain measures of the efficiency and use of the smartphone in everyday situations once the learning phase ended, daily self-reports were used again. The daily self-reports were very similar to the baseline measures (one-page table).

To measure the use of ARCUS, ND had to document the number of names he could not retrieve, the number of times ARCUS was used, the number of successful name retrievals using ARCUS and the number of times he still referred to his paper notebook. Follow-up measures were taken daily, from the end of the intervention to 10 weeks post-intervention.

Data Analyses

Results are based on ND's normal work days (Monday to Thursday) and included the days he met at least one person whose name could not be retrieved. The days ND did not have to look for a name (e.g., he worked alone all day or did not have difficulty finding the names of people he met that day) were removed from analyses. Therefore, 5 days were included at baseline, 8 days at intervention and 29 days at follow-up.

First, visual analyses of graph data were used to compare the tendency to compensate from baseline, to intervention, to follow-up. Visual analyses were also used to contrast the use of ARCUS and the paper notebook.

Non-parametric tests, such as the Kruskal-Wallis, could not be used to compare the three phases of the experiment since the homogeneity of variance assumption was not met. The difficulty dealing with the variance is discussed later in the results section.

Results

Visual Analysis

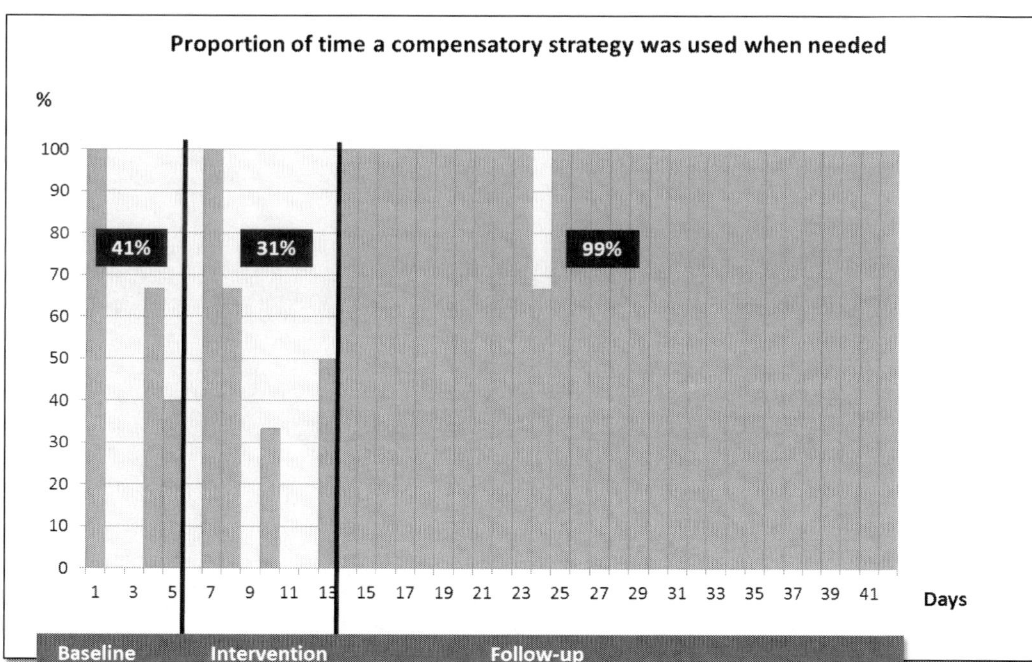

Figure 2. Proportion of time a compensatory strategy was used when needed.

The first goal of Study 1 was to measure changes in the general tendency to compensate when ARCUS was added to the paper notebook as a second possible strategy. Visual analysis of the graph data shows that the general tendency to use a compensatory strategy when needed (i.e. number of times a compensatory strategy was used each time a name was not retrieved) increased sharply from baseline to post-intervention (see Figure 2).

At baseline, when only the paper notebook was available, ND compensated 41% of the time (mean). During the intervention, when the paper notebook and ARCUS were available, and when a therapist accompanied ND to work to teach him now to use ARCUS, ND compensated 31% (mean) of the time he met a person whose name he could not recall. Post-intervention, when the paper notebook and ARCUS were both available and training was finished, ND compensated 99% (mean) of the time. Other than the sharp increase in the use of compensatory strategies, visual analysis of the graph data also shows a clear stabilization of compensation with less fluctuation in its use. This stabilization is also reflected in the standard deviation that decreases from phase to phase (SD baseline = 43%, SD intervention = 38%, SD follow-up = 6%). Compared to baseline and intervention, follow-up was the only time period where at least one compensatory strategy was used each day a name could not be retrieved.

The second goal of Study 1 was to compare use of the paper notebook and ARCUS. The contrasted use of the paper notebook and ARCUS for retrieving people's names is shown in Figure 3.

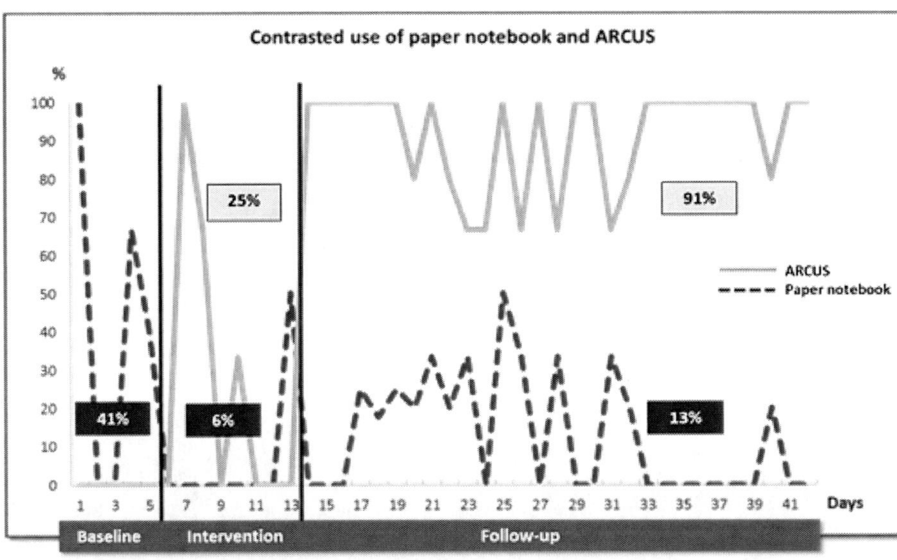

Figure 3. Contrasted use of paper notebook and ARCUS.

Visual analysis of the graph data shows that the tendency to use the paper notebook decreased from baseline to intervention/follow-up (mean (SD): 41% at baseline (43), 6% at intervention (17), 13% at follow-up (15). Visual analysis also shows an increase in the tendency to use the smartphone (ARCUS) from intervention to follow-up (mean (SD): 25% at intervention (38), 91% at follow-up (13).

Compared to the paper notebook, visual analysis shows that the smartphone (ARCUS) was the preferred compensatory strategy during intervention and follow-up, although the paper notebook was still available to ND. In fact, he resorted to it when he could not previously find a name in ARCUS, which happened, for example, when a name was not already programmed in the smartphone or when surface dysgraphia led to an ineffective search on the smartphone.

The third goal of Study 1 was to measure the effectiveness of ARCUS. The proportion of times ND completed an efficient search when he used ARCUS was measured (intervention: mean = 93%, SD = 11%, range = 80-100%; follow-up: mean = 90%, SD = 19%, range = 50-100%) and was considered satisfactory.

The variance issue. At first, non-parametric analyses, such as the Kruskal-Wallis test, and effect sizes (Beeson and Robey, 2006) were planned to statistically support the visual analysis comparison between the three phases of the study. However, the homogeneity of variance assumption could not be met, due to the large variance at baseline and intervention compared to maintenance (e.g., Figure 2: SD at baseline = 43%, SD at intervention = 36%, SD at maintenance = 6%). On these points, the variance may seem to compromise the data analysis and interpretation of the results. However, the lack of homogeneity of variance was a predictable and almost favorable issue in this study. Indeed, the uneven and fickle use of the paper notebook was a concern for ND before the study. In fact, he used his paper notebook when it was possible and the strategy was not applied evenly from day to day, leading to a statistical large variance at baseline and to a behavioral large variability in his tendency to compensate. The introduction of ARCUS was projected as a way to decrease this great variability in the use of compensatory strategies. In fact, this is what happened and the variance sharply decreased after intervention, leading to steadier use of compensatory strategies. Thus, the lack of homogeneity of variance supports and illustrates our first aim to help ND retrieve names.

Study 2. Impaired Word Comprehension and Anomia: Use of the Paper Dictionary and the Internet

An AB design was used. The procedure included (A) baseline measures and (B) introduction of the Internet on the smartphone as a compensatory strategy, plus follow-up measures.

(A) Baseline. Before providing the Internet, ND was asked to complete a daily self-report (one-page table) for one week to document the use of a paper dictionary. He was asked to note the number of times he used a dictionary and the number of times the search was efficient.

(B) Introduction of the Internet on the smartphone and follow-up measures. As for ARCUS, the Sohlberg and Mateer (1989) method was used with ND. Only one intensive 2-hour session was needed to teach him how to search the Internet (acquisition and application). During the training, the use of search engines or free encyclopaedias available on Internet was learned. ND was trained to use two specific websites where he could find semantic information (Wikipedia) or pictures of words (Google Image). At the end of this session, ND was able to use both websites. Because ND could also take advantage of the "standard" uses of the smartphone (i.e. making phone calls or sending text messages), another 2-hour session was given to teach him these functionalities. No measures were performed on these functionalities because the intervention did not target them.

To obtain measures of the efficiency and use of the Internet with the smartphone in everyday situations, daily self-reports, similar to the baseline measures, were again used. To measure use of the Internet, ND had to document the number of times he used the smartphone to search for information about a word, the efficiency of the search and the ease of obtaining the desired information on a five-point Likert scale (1 = very easy, 5 = very difficult).

Follow-up measures were taken daily, from the end of the baseline measures to 10 weeks post-introduction of the smartphone.

Data Analysis

Results were originally based on 83 consecutive days. Four days were removed because the Internet was out of service for technical difficulties. Another 4 days were removed from the analysis because ND did not report his use of the phone. Thus, a total of 75 days were included in the data analyses. Only visual analysis and raw data were used for Study 2. Indeed, it was almost impossible to collect the number of times a word was not understood or was not found in memory so that the reported measures did not allow us to calculate the real need for compensation of comprehension deficit and anomia. Therefore, no percentage of compensation (e.g., number of times a dictionary was used each time a word was not understood) could be calculated.

Results

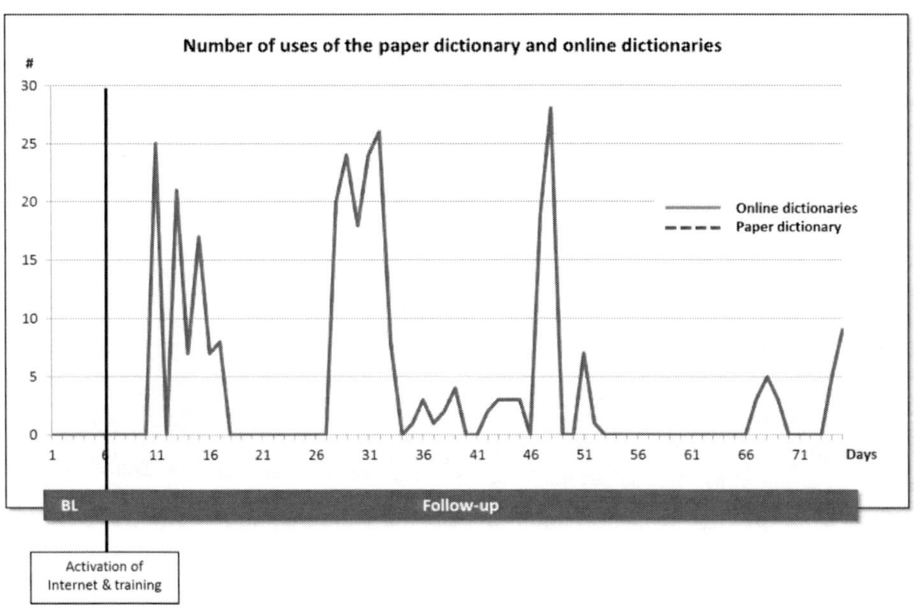

Figure 4. Number of uses of the paper dictionary and online dictionaries.

In Study 2, aimed at compensating for word comprehension and naming difficulties, the first goal was to measure use of the smartphone to search the Internet and the second goal was to compare use of the Internet and the paper dictionary.

Figure 4 shows the number of times ND used the paper dictionary (at baseline) and the Internet on the smartphone (follow-up) to search for semantic information.

ND reported that he rarely referred to the paper dictionary before the study. Moreover, no search in the paper dictionary was noted at baseline or during follow-up. The fluctuation in use of the Internet during the post-intervention period (range = 0-28) reflected ND's needs for semantic information. For example, he frequently used the Internet on the days he had to prepare activities for the residents (e.g., crosswords). Visual analysis of the graph data demonstrates that ND clearly tended to use Internet dictionaries more than the paper dictionary. However, this tendency fluctuated from day to day. The third goal of Study 2 was to measure the ease and effectiveness of using the smartphone to search the Internet. The proportion of times ND performed an efficient search in the Internet dictionaries was therefore calculated. The mean percentage was 90% (SD =13%, range = 66-100%, mode = 100%). The effectiveness of Internet searches is considered satisfactory. The ease of using the Internet was also reported by ND on a five-point Likert scale (1 = very easy, 5 = very difficult). The mean was 2 and the range was 2 to 3. Therefore, ND considered searching the Internet on the smartphone easy.

Discussion

The main goal of this study was to investigate the effectiveness of an ecological intervention in SD, focusing on needs in ADL. This goal was pursued using compensation strategies supported by new technologies. More specifically, the objectives of this case study were to measure the effectiveness of a smartphone in finding the names of people met at work (Study 1), and to find semantic information essential to comprehension and naming (Study 2). The results showed a sharp increase in the general tendency to compensate for people's name finding difficulties (Study 1) after the introduction of the smartphone. A large general preference for the smartphone (ARCUS) over the paper notebook to compensate for name finding difficulties was also found, and the effectiveness of the smartphone was very satisfactory. Four months after the end of the study, ND reported that he had completely dropped the paper notebook and exclusively used the smartphone with ARCUS. The results also showed that ND referred more to Internet dictionaries than to the paper dictionary to find semantic information (Study 2). The effectiveness of the Internet searches and the ease of searching were also very satisfactory. Therefore, the goals of this case study were considered to be largely achieved.

ND's use of a compensation strategy for retrieving people's names after the introduction of ARCUS was constant and efficient. It may have been enhanced by the ease of use of the smartphone and the ARCUS application. The smartphone provides a fast, efficient, portable, accessible and non-stigmatizing way to compensate for the difficulty. In contrast, the paper notebook, which was not used systematically by ND at baseline, is cumbersome, certainly not as mobile as the smartphone, and more stigmatizing (Rouleau et al., 2006). Compared to ARCUS, the compensation strategy for retrieving semantic information with the Internet search engine and free applications fluctuated more over time. This fluctuation probably reflects the variability in ND's needs for semantic information. However, those needs were not measured specifically in our study.

Nonetheless, these results are generally in line with what has been observed in Alzheimer Disease (AD), in which the use of compensation strategies has been more frequently documented. Quittre et al. (2009) used a combination of a mobile phone and a calendar with a person living with AD to improve spatiotemporal orientation and the results were successful. Lekeu et al. (2002) also showed an improvement in autonomy in ADL by training two persons in the early stage of AD to use a mobile phone. Imbeault et al. (2011) also reported an improvement in time management (e.g. appointments) for a person living with AD when using an electronic organizer. Our study thus confirms that a compensation strategy can be successfully used in dementia, when it is chosen according to the person's needs and when its use is taught with appropriate learning methods (Jacquemin, 2009). However, our results take this conclusion further since they were obtained for the first time with a person suffering from SD and in a working environment. In AD as well as in SD, the success of the intervention and compensation strategy seems to rely, at least in part, on preserved cognitive functions. Indeed, learning to use the new compensatory strategy could have relied on preserved procedural memory in AD (Beatty et al., 1994) and it could be hypothesized that new learning for ND also relied on this type of long term memory to quickly learn how to use the device and use it spontaneously when appropriate. In comparison to people living with AD, ND could also have relied on preserved episodic memory to create and use his personal clues to retrieve people's names.

Although the study focused on ND's needs at work (from Monday to Thursday), he also used ARCUS on Friday and over the weekend. This generalization of the compensation strategy across different real-life circumstances is noteworthy. In language-based therapy for people living with SD, when generalization concerns spontaneous improvement of untreated associated concepts (i.e. concepts sharing attributes with the concepts treated), results are usually very limited (for a review see Croot et al., 2009). This kind of generalization relies on the damaged semantic memory network and is quite difficult to obtain (Lambon Ralph and Patterson, 2008). However, when generalization relates instead to the application of a compensation strategy in appropriate contexts, people living with SD can rely on their preserved non-verbal episodic and procedural memory abilities (Adlam, Patterson, and Hodges, 2009; Graham, Kropelnicki, Goldman, and Hodges, 2003; Graham and Hodges, 1997) to support efficient use of the strategy.

Although ND's results are promising, they should be interpreted with caution. The sharp increase in the propensity to use the compensation device could have been influenced by other mediator variables, such as a sudden awareness that compensation is useful or a desire to please the experimenter (social desirability). However, ND's use of his smartphone over the weekend suggests that he enjoyed it and perceived its usefulness. Also, ND was already familiar with new technologies, and a question remains concerning the use of new technologies in the older adult population with little or no experience with them. However, as pointed out by Varley (2011), who debated the use of computers in aphasia therapy, good software design and engineering can make the use of new technologies very accessible. The application created for ND was designed to be easy to use. For example, very few windows were needed to search for a name in ARCUS. Moreover, in the application we used the vocabulary and wordings that ND used in his paper notebook, which were highly significant to him. A relevant training program (e.g., Sohlberg and Mateer, 1989) like the one used with ND can also lead to efficient learning of new procedures (e.g., use of a smartphone) even with people suffering from severe amnesia (Lekeu et al., 2002; Imbeault et al., 2011). Therefore, good software design and a relevant training program, properly combined with preserved cognitive functions, should be considered when using technology with people suffering from neurodegenerative disorders. Moreover, this alleged technological barrier will probably disappear in the coming years, with technologies becoming more and more present in everyone's everyday life. Finally, our study explored a specific intervention for one person in particular and it allowed us to create an application specifically designed for his needs. However, as only one case was studied, there is a need to replicate these results before generalization to the SD population. We are also interested in pursuing this research and looking at changes in use of the smartphone with the progression of the disease, i.e. how the continuing decline of semantic memory and other cognitive functions in the later stages of SD quantitatively and qualitatively affect the use of the compensatory strategy.

Overall, this case study suggests the clinical relevance of using an ecological intervention in the management of SD, focusing on the specific needs of people living with SD and on the use of compensation devices. Unlike other therapy studies where improving language performance was the main target (e.g., Funnell, 1995; Graham et al., 2001; Jokel et al., 2002, 2006; Snowden and Neary, 2002; Henry et al., 2008; Bier et al., 2009; Heredia et al., 2009), this study explored an ecological intervention approach aimed at helping people compensate for their deficits in ADL. The differences between classic language therapy and ecological interventions in SD is that the first focused on relearning one name/concept at a time during therapies whereas the second focused on compensating for every name/concept every time it is needed in ADL. The smartphone is a promising way to achieve this type of compensation. Replication of the present study with more people living with SD would be of great interest in order to generalize the results.

Acknowledgments

The authors would like to thank ND and his wife for participating in this study.

Funding

The first author was supported by a Vanier Canada Graduate Scholarship (Canadian Institutes of Health Research).

References

Adlam, A. L., Patterson, K., and Hodges, J. R. (2009). "I remember it as if it were yesterday": memory for recent events in patients with semantic dementia. *Neuropsychologia, 47*, 1344-1351.

Barbeau, E., Tramoni, E., Joubert, S., Mancini, J., Ceccaldi, M., and Poncet, M. (2004). Évaluation de la mémoire de reconnaissance visuelle : normalisation d'une nouvelle épreuve en choix forcé (DMS48) et utilité en neuropsychologie clinique. In M. Van der

Linden, S. Adam, A. Agniel, et les membres du GREMEM (Eds.), *L'évaluation des troubles de la mémoire* (pp. 85-101). Marseille, France: Solal.

Beatty, W. W., Winn, P., Adams, R. L., Allen, E. W., Wilson, D. A., Prince, J. R., Olson, K. A., et al. (1994). Preserved cognitive skills in dementia of the Alzheimer type. *Archives of Neurology, 51,* 1040-1046.

Beeson, P. M., and Robey, R. R. (2006). Evaluating single-subject treatment research: lessons learned from the aphasia literature. *Neuropsychology Review, 16,* 161-169.

Bier, N., and Macoir, J. (2010). How to make a spaghetti sauce with a dozen small things that I cannot name: A review of the impact of semantic memory deficits on everyday action. *Journal of Clinical and Experimental Neuropsychology, 32*, 201-211.

Bier, N., Macoir, J., Gagnon, L., Van der Linden, M., Louveaux, S., and Desrosiers, J. (2009). Known, lost, and recovered: Efficacy of formal-semantic therapy and spaced retrieval method in a case of semantic dementia. *Aphasiology, 22,* 210-235.

Bier, N., Macoir, J., and Joubert, S. (2011). Cooking "Shrimp à la Créole": A pilot study of an ecological rehabilitation in semantic dementia. *Neuropsychological Rehabilitation, 21,* 455-483.

Bozeat, S., Lambon Ralph, M. A., Patterson, K., and Hodges, J. R. (2002). When objects lose their meaning: What happens to their use? *Cognitive, Affective and Behavioral neuroscience, 2,* 236-251.

Bozeat, S., Patterson, K., and Hodges, J. (2004). Relearning object use in semantic dementia. *Neuropsychological Rehabilitation, 14*, 351-363.

Breedin, S. D., Saffran, E. M., and Coslett, H. B. (1994). Reversal of the concreteness effect in a patient with semantic dementia. *Cognitive Neuropsychology, 11,* 617-660.

Burgess, P. W. and Shallice, T. (1997). The Hayling and Brixton Tests. Bury St. Edmunds, UK: Thames Valley Test Company.

Burrell, J. R., and Hodges, J. R. (2010). From FUS to Fibs: What's new in frontotemporal dementia? *Journal of Alzheimer's Disease, 21,* 349-360.

Croot, K., Nickels, L., Laurence, F., and Manning, M. (2009). Impairment- and activity/participation-directed interventions in progressive language impairment: Clinical and theoretical issues. *Aphasiology, 23,* 125-160.

Delis, D. C., Kaplan, E., and Kramer, J. H. (2001). *Delis-Kaplan Executive Function System (D-KEFS).* San Antonio, TX: The Psychological Corporation.

Dewar, B.-K., Patterson, K., Wilson, B. A., and Graham, K. S. (2009). Re-acquisition of person knowledge in semantic memory disorders. *Neuropsychological Rehabilitation, 19,* 383-421.

Frattali, C. (2004). An errorless learning approach to treating dysnomia in frontotemporal dementia. *Journal of Medical Speech-Language Pathology, 12,* 11-24.

Funnell, E. (1995). A case of forgotten knowledge. In R. Campbell and M. Conway (Eds.), *Broken memories: Case studies in memory impairment.* (pp. 225-236). Oxford, UK: Blackwell.

Golden, J. C. (1978). Stroop color and word test. Chicago, IL: Stoelting Co.

Gorno-Tempini, M. L., Hillis, A. E., Weintraub, S., Kertesz, A., Mendez, M., Cappa, S. F., Ogar, J. M., et al. (2011). Classification of primary progressive aphasia and its variants. *Neurology, 76,* 1006-1014.

Graham, K. S., and Hodges, J. R. (1997). Differentiating the roles of the hippocampal complex and the neocortex in long-term memory storage; evidence from the study of semantic dementia and Alzheimer's disease. *Neuropsychology, 11,* 77-89.

Graham, K. S., Kropelnicki, A., Goldman, W. P., and Hodges, J. H. (2003). Two further investigations of autobiographical memory in semantic dementia. *Cortex, 39,* 729-750.

Graham, K. S., Patterson, K., Pratt, K. H., and Hodges, J. R. (1999). Relearning and subsequent forgetting of semantic category exemplars in a case of semantic dementia. *Neuropsychology, 13,* 359-380.

Graham, K. S., Patterson, K., Pratt, K. H., and Hodges, J. R. (2001). Can repeated exposure to "forgotten" vocabulary help alleviate word-finding difficulties in semantic dementia? An illustrative case study. *Neuropsychological Rehabilitation, 11,* 429-454.

Hamanaka, T., Matsui, A., Yoshida, S., Nakanishi, M., Fujita, K., and Banno, T. (1996). Cerebral laterality and category-specificity in cases of semantic memory impairment with PET-findings and associated with identification amnesia for familiar persons. *Brain and Cognition, 30,* 368-372.

Henry, M. L., Besson, P. M., and Rapcsak, S. Z. (2008). Treatment for anomia in semantic dementia. *Seminars in Speech and Language, 29,* 60-70.

Heredia, C. G. Sage, K., Lambon Ralph, M. A., and Berthier, M. L. (2009). Relearning and retention of verbal labels in a case of semantic dementia. *Aphasiology, 23,* 192-209.

Hodges, J. R., Bozeat, S., Lambon Ralph, M. A., Patterson, K., and Spatt, J. (2000). The role of conceptual knowledge in object use: Evidence from semantic dementia. *Brain, 123,* 1913-1925.

Hodges, J. R., and Graham, K. S. (1998). A reversal of the temporal gradient for famous person knowledge in semantic dementia: Implications for the neural organisation of long-term memory. *Neuropsychologia, 36,* 803-825.

Hodges, J. R., Graham, N., and Patterson, K. (1995). Charting the progression in semantic dementia: Implications for the organisation of semantic memory. *Memory, 3,* 463-495.

Hodges, J. R., Patterson, K., Oxbury, S., and Funnell, E. (1992). Semantic dementia: progressive fluent aphasia with temporal lobe atrophy. *Brain, 115,* 1783-1806.

Hodges, J. R, Patterson, K., and Tyler, L. K. (1994). Loss of semantic memory: implications for the modularity of mind. *Cognitive Neuropsychology, 11,* 505-542.

Howard, D., and Patterson, K. (1992). *The Pyramids and Palm Trees Test: A test for semantic access from words and pictures.* Bury St Edmunds, UK : Thames Valley Test Company.

Imbeault, H., Pigot, H., Bier, N., Gagnon, L., Giroux, S., Marcotte, N., and Fülöp, T. (2011). Interdisciplinary design of an electronic organizer for persons with Alzheimer's disease. In B. Abdulrazak et al. (Eds.), *ICOST 2011, LNCS 6719* (pp. 137-144).

Jacquemin, A. (2009). Strategy and methods of cognitive rehabilitation in patients with Alzheimer's disease or other dementia. *Psychologie et Neuropsychiatrie du Vieillissement, 7,* 265-273.

Joanette, Y., Ska, B., Belleville, S., Lecours, A.R., Peretz, I., and Poissant, A. (1995). Évaluation neuropsychologique dans la démence de type Alzheimer: un compromis optimal. *L'année gérontologique, 3,* 69-83.

Jokel, R., Rochon, E., and Leonard, C. (2002). Therapy for anomia in semantic dementia. *Brain and Cognition, 49,* 241-244.

Jokel, R., Rochon, E., and Leonard, C. (2006). Treating anomia in semantic dementia: Improvement, maintenance, or both? *Neuropsychological Rehabilitation, 16,* 241-256.

Jokel, R., Cupit, J., Rochon, E. A., and Graham, N. L. (2007). Errorless re-training in semantic dementia using MossTalk Words. *Brain and Language, 103,* 248-249.

Jokel, R., Rochon, E., and Anderson, N. D. (2010). Errorless learning of computer-generated words in a patient with semantic dementia. *Neuropsychological Rehabilitation, 20,* 16-41.

Kashibayashi, T., Ikeda, M., Komori, K., Shinagawa, S., Shimizu, H., Toyota, Y., et al., (2010). Transition of distinctive symptoms of semantic dementia during longitudinal clinical observation.*Dementia and geriatric cognitive disorders, 29,* 224-232.

Lambon Ralph, M. A., and Patterson, K. (2008). Generalization and differentiation in semantic memory: Insights from semantic dementia. *Annals of the New York Academy of Sciences, 1124,* 61-76.

Lekeu, F., Wojtasik, V., Van der Linden, M., and Salmon, E. (2002). Training early Alzheimer patients to use a mobile phone. *Acta Neurologica Belgica, 102*, 114-121.

Macoir, J., Beaudoin, C., and Bluteau, J. (2008). *Le test de dénomination d'images de Québec: TDQ-60.* Université Laval: Québec.

Macoir, J., Gauthier, S., and Jean, C. (2005). *Batterie d'Évaluation Cognitive du Langage chez l'Adulte (BECLA).* Université Laval: Québec.

Mioshi, E., and Hodges, J. R. (2009). Rate of change of functional abilities in frontotemporal dementia. *Dementia and Geriatric Cognitive Disorders, 28,* 419-426.

Mioshi, E., Kipps, C. M., Dawson, K., Mitchell, J., Graham, A., and Hodges, J. R. (2007). Activities of daily living in frontotemporal dementia and Alzheimer disease. *Neurology, 68,* 2077-2084.

Neary, D., Snowden, J. S., Gustafson, L., Passant, U., Stuss, D., Black, S. et al. (1998). Frontotemporal lobar degeneration: A consensus on clinical diagnostic criteria. *Neurology, 51,* 1546-1554.

Nespoulous, J-L., Lecours, A. R., Lafond, D., Lemay, A., Puel, M., Joanette, Y., et al. (1992). *Protocole Montréal-Toulouse d'examen linguistique de l'aphasie. MT-86 Module Standard Initial: M1 [Montréal-Toulouse Protocole of Linguistic Evaluation of Aphasia. MT-86 Initial Standard Module: M1]. (2nd ed. revised by Renée Béland and Francine Giroux).* Isbergues, France: L'Ortho-Édition.

Ottenbacher, K. (1986). *Evaluating clinical change: Strategies for occupational and physical therapists.* Baltimore, MD: Williams and Wilkins.

Quittre, A., Adam, S., Olivier, C., and Salmon, E. (2009). Maintien d'une orientation spatio-temporelle chez une patiente Alzheimer: Utilisation conjointe d'un agenda et d'un téléphone portable. In S. Adam, P. Allain, G. Aubin and F. Coyette (Eds.), *Actualités en rééducation neuropsychologique: Études de cas* (pp. 333-365). Marseille, France: Solar.

Reitan, R.M. (1958). Validity of the Trail Making Test as an indicator of organic brain damage. *Perceptual and Motor Skills, 8,* 271-276.

Riddoch, M. J., and Humphreys, G. W. (1993). *The Birmingham Object Recognition Battery.* Hove, UK: Lawrence Erlbaum Associates Ltd.

Robinson, S., Druks, J., Hodges, J., and Garrard, P. (2009). The treatment of object naming, definition, and object use in semantic dementia: The effectiveness of errorless learning. *Aphasiology, 23,* 749-775.

Rouleau, I., Brière, S., Imbeault, H., Laflamme, K., and Lefèbvre, A.A. (2006). Compensation des troubles de la mémoire prospective par l'utilisation du carnet de mémoire. *Revue Québécoise de Psychologie, 27,* 87-104.

Shinagawa, S., Ikeda, M., Fukuhara, R., and Tanabe, H. (2006). Initial symptoms in frontotemporal dementia compared with Alzheimer's disease. *Dementia and Geriatric Cognitive Disorders, 21,* 74-80.

Snowden, J., Griffiths, H., and Neary, D. (1994). Semantic dementia: Autobiographical contribution to preservation of meaning. *Cognitive Neuropsychology, 11,* 265-288.

Snowden, J. S., Bathgate, D., Varma, A., Blackshaw, A., Gibbons, Z. C., and Neary, D. (2001). Distinct behavioural profiles in frontotemporal dementia and semantic dementia. *Journal of Neurology, Neurosurgery and Psychiatry, 70,* 323-332.

Snowden, J. S., and Neary, D. (2002). Relearning of verbal labels in semantic dementia. *Neuropsychologia, 40,* 1715-1728.

Sohlberg, M. M., and Mateer, C. A. (1989). Training use of compensatory memory books: a three-stage behavioral approach. *Journal of Clinical and Experimental Neuropsychology, 11,* 871-891.

Svoboda, E., and Richards, B. (2009). Compensating for anterograde amnesia: A new training method that capitalizes on emerging smartphone technologies. *Journal of the International Neuropsychological Society, 15,* 629-638.

Varley, R. (2011). Rethinking aphasia therapy: A neuroscience perspective. *International Journal of Speech-Language Pathology, 13,* 11-20.

Wilson, B. A. (1987). Single-case experimental designs in neuropsychological rehabilitation. *Journal of Clinical and Experimental Neuropsychology, 9,* 527-544.

In: Non-Pharmacological Therapies ...
Editor: Elisabetta Farina

ISBN: 978-1-63321-860-4

Chapter 9

Effectiveness (or Not?) of Cognitive Rehabilitation in a Person with Semantic Dementia

Fabiana Villanelli*[*1], Annamaria Russo[2], Raffaello Nemni[1] and Elisabetta Farina[1]
[1]Neurorehabilitation Unit, IRCCS "S. Maria Nascente",
Don Gnocchi Foundation, Milan, Italy
[2]Neurological Unit, Humanitas Gavazzeni, Bergamo, Italy

Abstract

We tested the possible efficacy of relearning ecologically relevant information and its maintenance in Marian, a person affected by Semantic Dementia (SD).

In Phase 1, 20 images, belonging to two different categories of objects (vegetables and fruit), have been chosen among the ones Marian did not recognize: in each category, 5 have been used for the 2 month training (twice a week) with explicit and implicit memory techniques while the other 5 haven't. Statistical analysis comparing *trained-not trained* words at the end of the rehabilitation period was not significant, even if a slightly better performance in rehabilitated words was evident. At 6 months follow-up no training gain was evident.

In Phase 2, we performed a repeated baseline assessment and then we introduced a photo-vocabulary, which included 14 relatives' names. At baseline, Marian constantly denominated 1 relative only. In this second phase, Marian both followed structured rehabilitation sessions and rehearsed face-name associations at home. After two months Marian named 8/14 relatives (14/14 after phonemic cue). At 6 months follow-up, she spontaneously named 11/14 relatives' names (14/14 after phonemic cue).

In the second training phase, Marian showed a clearer improvement. This better result could depend on the fact that relatives' identification was less affected than

[*] Corresponding Author: Fabiana Villanelli, Neurorehabilitation Unit, IRCCS "Santa Maria Nascente", Fondazione Don Gnocchi, Via Capecelatro 66, 20148 Milano, Italy, tel ++39-02-40308280, fax ++39-02-40308290, f.villanelli@alice.it

identification of different kinds of food, or on the intensiveness of training or on Marian's better motivation.

The progression of the disease, however, stopped us from further treating Marian. Therefore, as shown by other Authors, a cognitive rehabilitation training based on relearning with explicit and implicit memory techniques seems to show a limited effectiveness in SD.

Keywords: Semantic Dementia (SD), cognitive rehabilitation in dementia, explicit and implicit memory techniques, rehabilitation at home by relatives

Introduction

Semantic Dementia (SD) is one of the main clinical variants of frontotemporal lobar degeneration (FTLD), which includes also progressive non-fluent aphasia (PNFA) and frontotemporal dementia - frontal variant (fv-FTD). The typical reduction of the expressive vocabulary is the most prominent early feature of SD .

People with SD face a progressive loss of semantic information about people, objects, facts and words; in particular, the language disorder – with insidious onset and gradual progression - is characterized by fluent and empty spontaneous speech, loss of word meaning (impaired naming and comprehension), semantic paraphasias; furthermore, a perceptual disorder is present, characterized by prosopoagnosia (impaired recognition of identity of familiar faces) and/or associative agnosia (impaired recognition of object identity), while perceptual matching and drawing reproduction, single-word repetition and ability to read aloud and write ortographically regular words from dictation are preserved (Neary, 1999).

People with SD may have a non-specific memory impairment, but this does not reflect a true amnesia: in contrast with Alzheimer Disease (AD), memory for recent daily events is relatively preserved; consequently, people affected by SD are not significantly impaired in Activities of Daily Living in the first phases of the disease, in spite of the significant language involvement (Hodges and Patterson, 2007).

Furthermore, Graham et al. (2003) have demonstrated a reverse temporal gradient on tests of autobiographical memory in SD, which is in contrast with other degenerative dementias, such as Alzheimer's Disease. This result may be explained by considering that the hippocampal complex and the temporal neocortex play separate yet interactive roles in the acquisition and maintenance of autobiographical and semantic knowledge (Takashima et al., 2009). According to this theory, although our long-term memory is ultimately represented in neocortical regions, the hippocampus and related structures play a vital role in the initial phase of memory representation. On this basis, as long as the hippocampal system is relatively intact, people with SD should be capable of at least some forms of new learning.

Relearning ecologically relevant information could positively impact on quality of life of people with SD. As an example, the profound word-finding and comprehension difficulties experienced by persons affected by SD – particularly the inability to remember the names of people – diminish their social confidence and often lead them and their spouses to isolation.

Rehabilitation interventions proposed for people with SD have been mainly focused in improving naming (e.g. Graham et al., 1999, 2001; Croot et al., 2009; Dressel et al., 2010), or in the use of objects (e.g. Bozeat et al., 2004; Robinson et al., 2009). However, even if some language improvement has been demonstrated, it is often slight and limited to "trained" items associated with specific temporo-spatial contexts and it vanishes rapidly; see for a review (Henry et al., 2008). More rarely Authors have reported more encouraging results (Jokel et al., 2007, 2010; Graham et al., 1999).

In order to improve naming, several techniques have been proposed, from the simple presentation of pictures with a brief description of the object (Jokel et al, 2006) to the use of complex phonological and semantic cueing hierarchies (Dressel et al., 2010), to protocols incorporating errorless learning principles (Frattali, 2004; Jokel et al., 2010).

Testing the possible efficacy of an 'ecologically relevant information' re-learning program (i.e. naming of common items, name-face association for relatives) together with the maintenance of the same information in a person affected by SD were the objectives of the present study.

Case Report

Marian is a 67 years old woman who - for 4 years – has shown difficulties in associating names with objects and people and does not remember the significance of many words frequently used (for example "carrot", "phrase", "count"). The first time she came to our attention, her episodic memory was only slightly compromised in the ecologic field: sometimes she did not remember the localization of objects and needed to be accompanied at least once or twice to unknown places before she could orient herself. Daily living activities were preserved: she continued to be a good cook and she could still and efficiently take care of her own house and her daughter's.

Objectively she presented fluent and logorrheic speech, with anomias and difficulties in its construction; she did not remember the meaning of many words, both concrete and abstract, in particular about animal, fruit and vegetable categories

She completed some diagnostic instrumental and laboratory assessments: blood exams were normal; brain Magnetic Resonance Imaging showed an evident left insular-temporal atrophy, associated with mild cortical-subcortical anterior-temporal and mesial hyperintensity (T2), clear enlargement of temporal horn of left lateral ventricle, and a certain degree of hippocampal atrophy (See Figure 1). SPECT showed prefrontal and left medial-temporal hypoperfusion.

At neuropsychological assessment Marian showed: comprehension deficit in the Token test (she confused circles and squares), misunderstanding of commonly used words, deficits in picture naming (with clear dissociation between living and not-living in a not structured questionnaire, but not in a semantic memory questionnaire), dramatic impairment in naming personalities (even when she recognized them, information about life and activities appeared scanty and imprecise), in associating stimuli belonging to the same semantic category (but perceptively different) and in discrimination between real and chimeric figures (especially if characterized by great perceptual complexity).

Semantic fluency appeared markedly compromised, while phonologic fluency was profusely normal. Verbal learning was impaired, but recall of visuospatial elements was preserved. MMSE score was 21/30.

Treatment (Cognitive Rehabilitation)

The purpose of cognitive rehabilitation in Marian was the direct re-learning of the name (along with some semantic and perceptive characteristics) of ecologically relevant items using phonemic and semantic cues, a verbal description of the object and possibly multisensorial stimulation (sight, tact, taste) to reactivate semantic connections; when this strategy appeared to fail, implicit memory techniques were used (that is:*vanishing cues forward* and *spaced retrieval* at 10", 20", 30", 1', 2' and 5', with application of *errorless learning*). Each phase of training lasted 2 months. Marian followed rehabilitation sessions twice a week. Every session lasted 45 minutes.

The study was approved by the local Ethical Committee. Marian gave her informed consent.

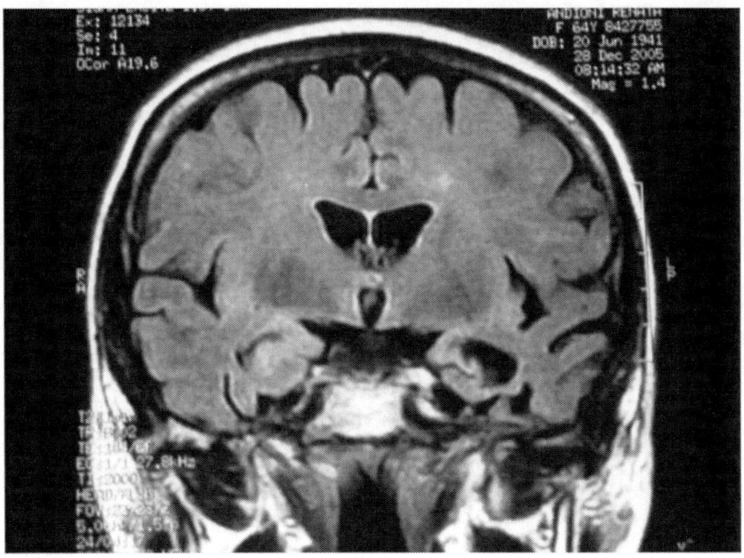

Figure 1. Marian's MRI scan.

Phase 1

Twenty images, belonging to two different categories of objects Marian was interested in (respectively, ten fruit and ten vegetables), were chosen among the ones she did not recognize in evaluation tests : in each category, 5 were trained, while the other 5 were not The purpose was a comparison of words *trained-not trained* at the end of the two months.

After eight sessions of 45 minutes, evaluation of *trained vs not trained* words showed a slight improvement in fruit and vegetables naming (with a better performance for the latter), but statistical analysis (*chi square*) of items *rehabilitated vs not rehabilitated* did not reach significance [Table 1]. When considering the results, please note that some data suggest better efficacy of phonemic cueing after training for people with SD (Mayberry et al., 2011).

Table 1. Phase 1: evaluation of *trained vs not trained* words (fruit, vegetables)

	vegetables	fruit
rehabilitated	spontaneously 3/5, after phonemic cue 4/5	spontaneously 1/5, after phonemic cue 5/5
not rehabilitated	spontaneously 1/5, after phonemic cue 4/5	spontaneously 1/5, after phonemic cue 2/5

Phase 2

For the rehabilitation program second phase – phase which had lasted for 2 months - we decided not to use a comparison between treated and not treated items, because we feared that the lack of significance of first phase results was due to some lack of power. We also decided to change the items of "nature" and we started choosing stimuli which could be more relevant for Marian from an emotional point of view. So, a different approach was used (see Clare, 1999, 2000).

We performed a repeated baseline assessment (4 times on a weekly basis). A photo-vocabulary including 14 names of relatives was introduced (It was not possible to get more relatives to train). At baseline, Marian constantly denominated only 1 relative (the same every time); we did not exclude this item from rehabilitation sessions so that the task was not so frustrating.

Rehabilitation sessions were performed using the same techniques as in Phase 1, but: then Marian had started using this material at home for her everyday training.

After the two-month training Marian named 8/14 relatives (14/14 after phonemic cue).

6-Months Follow up

We retested Marian's ability to denominate vegetables and fruit (phase 1) and relatives (phase 2). She spontaneously named 1/5 rehabilitated vegetables (4/5 after phonemic cue) and 0/5 fruit (4/5 after phonemic cue), 1/5 not rehabilitated vegetables (4/5 after phonemic cue) and 1/5 fruit (3/5 after phonemic cue). She spontaneously denominated 11/14 relatives' names (14/14 after phonemic cue). [Table 2]. At that time, Marian and her family showed great satisfaction about her training results. In the following months, however, further progression of the disease kept us from repeating a rehabilitation training because this had become too frustrating for Marian.

Table 2. 6-months follow-up

	vegetables	fruit	relatives
rehabilitated	spontaneously 1/5 after phonemic cue 4/5	spontaneously 0/5, after phonemic cue 4/5	11/14 spontaneously, 14/14 after phonemic cue
not rehabilitated	spontaneously 1/5 after phonemic cue 4/5	spontaneously 1/5, after phonemic cue 3/5	

Discussion

As far as the first phase of the training is concerned, statistical analysis (Chi-square P value) of rehabilitated *versus* not rehabilitated items (vegetables and fruit) was not significant, even if a slightly better performance in rehabilitated words was evident. This "negative" result could be due to the limited number of words taken into account. It must be also stressed that Marian did not train at home in this phase of the rehabilitation program. However these disappointing results could be also due to the limited efficacy of "traditional" relearning techniques in SD-people's rehabilitation.

In the second phase of training Marian showed a clearer improvement in naming relatives, suggesting at least a limited effectiveness of cognitive rehabilitation. In our opinion, this better result could depend on the association of training in hospital and at home. Intensiveness of training could be a critical point in assuring positive results (Graham et al., 1999; Jokel et al., 2006). However, the more positive results for relatives could also depend on Marian's better motivation. Studies have shown that, in people with Alzheimer disease, the emotional arousal enhances memory (Satler et al., 2007).

In fact, at 6 months follow-up Marian showed a worsening in naming but further improvement for relatives. This finding could mean that the affective value of these items had a positive influence even if we cannot exclude that relatives' identification was less affected than identification of food.

However, the progression of the disease stopped us from treating Marian further on. So, as shown by other Authors, a cognitive rehabilitation training based on relearning with explicit and implicit memory techniques appears to show a reduced effectiveness, limited to the first phase of the disease when a widespread brain atrophy is not present.

Alternative rehabilitation methods, based for example on external aids and/or implementation of technology resources, could be more promising in order to improve SD-people's quality of life. (Routhier et al, in press).

References

Bozeat, S., Patterson, K., and Hodges, J. (2004). Relearning object use in semantic dementia. *Neuropsychological Rehabilitation, 14*, 351-363.

Clare, L., Wilson, B.A, Breen, K., Hodges, J.R. (1999) Errorless learning of face-name association in early Alzheimer's disease. *Neurocase*, 5, 37-46

Clare, L., Wilson, B.A., Carter, G., Breen, K., Gosses, A., and Hodges, J.R. (2000). Intervening with everyday memory problems in dementia of Alzheimer type: an errorless learning approach. *J. Clin. Exp. Neuropsychol.*, 22(1),132-146.

Croot, K., Nickels, L., Laurence, F., and Manning, M. (2009). Impairment- and activity/participation-directed interventions in progressive language impairment: Clinical and theoretical issues. *Aphasiology, 23,* 125-160.

Dressel, K., Huber, W., Frings, L., Kümmerer, D., Saur, D., Mader, I.,

Hüll, M., Weiller, C., Abel. S. (2010): Model-oriented naming therapy in semantic dementia: A single-case fMRI study, *Aphasiology*, 24:12, 1537-1558. http://dx.doi.org/ 10.1080/02687038.2010.500567

Frattali, C. (2004). An errorless learning approach to treating dysnomia in frontotemporal dementia. *Journal of Medical Speech-Language Pathology, 12,* 11-24.

Graham, K. S., Patterson, K., Pratt, K. H., and Hodges, J. R. (2001). Can repeated exposure to "forgotten" vocabulary help alleviate word-finding difficulties in semantic dementia? An illustrative case study. *Neuropsychological Rehabilitation, 11,* 429-454.

Graham, K.S., Kropelnicki, A., Goldman, W.P, Hodges, J.R. (2003) Two further investigations of autobiographical memory in semantic dementia. Cortex. Sep-Dec;39(4-5), 729-50.

Graham, K.S., Patterson, K., Pratt, K.H., and Hodges, J.R. (1999). Relearning and subsequent forgetting of semantic category exemplars in a case of semantic dementia. *Neuropsychology*,13(3), 359-380.

Henry, M. L., Beeson, P. M., and Rapcsak, S. Z. (2008). Treatment for anomia in semantic dementia. *Seminars in Speech and Language, 29,* 60-70. doi:10.1055/s-2008-1061625.

Hodges, J.R., and Patterson, K. (2007). Semantic dementia: a unique clinicopathological syndrome. *Lancet Neurol*, 6, 1004-1014.

Jokel, R., Rochon, E., and Leonard, C. (2006). Treating anomia in semantic dementia: Improvement, maintenance, or both? *Neuropsychological Rehabilitation, 16,* 241-256.

Jokel, R., Cupit, J., Rochon, E. A., and Graham, N. L. (2007).Errorless re-training in semantic dementia using MossTalk Words. *Brain and Language, 103,* 248-249.

Jokel, R., Rochon, E., and Anderson, N. D. (2010).Errorless learning of computer generated words in a patient with semantic dementia.*Neuropsychological Rehabilitation, 20,* 16-41.

Mayberry, E.J, Sage, K., Ehsan, S. and Lambon Ralph, MA (2011): An emergent effect of phonemic cueing following relearning in semantic dementia. *Aphasiology,* 25:9, 1069-1077. http://dx.doi.org/10.1080/02687038.2011.575203.

Neary D. Overview of frontotemporal dementias and the consensus applied (1999). *Dement Geriatr Cogn Disord.* 10 Suppl 1, 6-9.

Robinson, S., Druks, J., Hodges, J., and Garrard, P. (2009). The treatment of object naming, definition, and object use in semantic dementia: The effectiveness of errorless learning. *Aphasiology, 23,* 749-775.

Routhier, S., Macoir, J. and Jacques, S. (in press) From smartphone to external semantic memory device: the use of new technologies to compensate for semantic deficits. *Non-pharmacological Therapies in Dementia*, in press.

Satler C., Garrido L.M., Sarmiento E.P., Leme S, Conde C., Tomaz C. (2007). Emotional arousal enhances declarative memory in patients with Alzheimer's disease. *Acta Neurol. Scand.* 116(6), 355-60.

Satler, C., Garrido, L. M., Sarmiento, E. P., Leme, S., Conde, C. and Tomaz, C. (2007), Emotional arousal enhances declarative memory in patients with Alzheimer's disease. *Acta Neurologica Scandinavica,* 116: 355–360. doi: 10.1111/j.1600-0404.2007.00897.

Saur, D., Mader, I., Hüll, M., Weiller, C. and Abel, S. (2010): Model-oriented naming

Takashima, A., Nieuwenhuis, I.L., Jensen, O., Talamin,i L.M., Rijpkema, M., Fernández G. (2009) Shift from hippocampal to neocortical centered retrieval network with consolidation. *J. Neurosci.* 2009 Aug 12;29(32):10087-93.

In: Non-Pharmacological Therapies ...
Editor: Elisabetta Farina
ISBN: 978-1-63321-860-4

Chapter 10

Impact of Non Pharmacologic Interventions on People with Dementia and Their Caregivers: A French Perspective

Florence Bonté*
FH Ste Marie, Paris, France

Abstract

The article briefly describes the characteristics of the geriatric care organization in France, and in particular the role of medium term Day care Hospital (DCH) and the personal experience of the Author in this setting. People with dementia admitted in medium term DCH are sent by specialists from the memory clinic, short term DCH, or general practitioners (GP), simply because of the need of rehabilitation or in case of a sudden crisis at home. In this setting, non-pharmacological therapies, among these Art and Music therapy, can be delivered to people with dementia, while their caregivers can receive information and support.

Keywords: Dementia, medium term day care hospital (DCH), non pharmacologic interventions, art therapy, music therapy

Introduction

Alzheimer's disease (AD) and related disorders are becoming increasingly common in older people, especially for those over 85, in France and elsewhere. In our country, the number of people with dementia is estimated at 1 million persons but 3 million people could be actually touched by the disease (INSEE, 2011).

* E-mail: fbonte@centresaintemarie.com

The course of the disease depends in part on the quality of care and the ability of carers. Most caregivers are family members, spouse or child; in the vast majority, women.

Caring for a person with dementia exposes caregivers to a high level of stress and can have psychiatric and physical effects; it's known that caregivers of people living with dementia - more often than caregivers of people with other diseases - suffer from anxiety, depression, addictions, and have an increased risk of mortality. The burden of caring for a person with dementia is financially, emotionally and physically significant, because of the social isolation and complex financial, legal and social decision making. Carers of people with dementia in the more advanced stages report that they often have only 2 hours a week, left for their personal pursuits (Aguglia, 2004).

Recent studies have shown that an overall management of the disease is able to contrast the cognitive decline. Pharmacological therapeutics are of modest efficacy and need to be combined with non-pharmacological therapies to offer a better response in people with dementia and to satisfy caregiver needs. Behavioral and psychological symptoms contribute to poor quality of life and high caregiver burden. The challenge for health care providers is to find safe and effective treatments for these symptoms. Non-pharmacological interventions are safer alternatives than pharmacotherapy, but too little is known about their effectiveness and tangible results. Few randomized, controlled trials are available and samples are often too small. However, multicomponent and psychoeducational interventions dedicated to the patient and the caregiver have shown a significant positive effect on caregivers. (Brodaty, 2003)

The impact of these interventions on caregivers of people with dementia is discussed in this article, making reference to our personal experience in a French geriatric Day Hospital setting. After an introduction on the organization of geriatric care in France and a description of the Geriatric Day Care Hospital setting, the main aspects of the support and treatment program offered will be discussed as well as their relevance based on the literature.

Characteristics of the Geriatric Care Organization in France

The pathways of Alzheimer's care can assist people with dementia and caregivers from diagnosis to treatment of complications or crisis' situations management (Volpe-Gillot, Bonté; 2008). There are two kinds of Day care Hospital (DCH) in France . Short term DCH are dedicated to diagnosis, while medium term DCH are dedicated to follow up and crisis resolution. People with dementia admitted in medium term DCH are sent by specialists from the memory clinic, short term DCH, or GP, simply because of the need of rehabilitation or in case of a sudden crisis at home. All people with dementia have a diagnosis, and are at mild to moderate stage of the disease. People with dementia have the right to stay at least 6 months in the unit with a stay of one or two days a week. The unit is composed by a multidisciplinary team headed by a geriatrician and proposes non-pharmacological interventions for people with dementia and caregivers after an individualized assessment of the whole situation of the person living with dementia. In our unit, the team, headed by the geriatrician, is composed by professionals working part-time: a nurse, a physiotherapist, a music-therapist, an art-therapist, an occupational therapist, a speech therapist, a psychologist, a social worker and a medical secretary. People with dementia are offered interventions, aimed to rehabilitation, resocialization, and to calm down BPSD. Caregivers are also involved in a psychoeducational program. During the stay, assessments are made to check the efficiency of the device. At the end of the stay, caregivers and people with dementia are referred towards respite care solutions and day care centers.

Medium term DCH are different from day care centers because they are not focused on respite, but on crisis resolution, intensive rehabilitation, and educational programs, provided by professionals of high level competence in dementia care.

The 2008-2012 Alzheimer Plan focused on improving the people with dementia and their caregivers' route, throughout the evolution of the pathology, by creating new and improved organizations and new kinds of businesses. The MAIAs (Maisons pour l'Autonomie et l'Integration des malades Alzheimer, "Houses for Autonomy and integration of Alzheimer patients") are spreading. Every MAIA is responsible for coordination of all actors in the same area. Improving vocational training of professional caregivers on the management of dementia was another important target. Thanks to this and as a consequence, a new job qualification has been created called: "Assistant en gérontologie": "Gerontology assistant". (www.plan-alzheimer.gouv.fr)

At the European level, the French Haute Autorité de Santé (HAS) is leading activities in a group named ALCOVE (ALzheimer COoperation and Valuation in Europe). "ALCOVE is a Joint Action between European Member States which aims to both improve the knowledge on dementia and its consequences and to promote the exchange of information to preserve health, quality of life, autonomy and dignity of caregivers and of people living with dementia in European Union Member States".

Caregiver Educational Program

Providing information and support is of great value to people with dementia and their families and caregivers. Caregivers express the need of more information on cognitive symptoms, on management of behavioral and psychological symptoms of dementia and on the expected clinical course of the disease. Caregivers express also the extreme need of constant emotional support. They wish to improve the quality of their daily care. Unfortunately, caregiving has negative consequences for caregivers' mental and physical health (Wu 1998; Yee, 1995). Anxiety and depression, overconsumption of drugs, such as psychotropic ones, are often found in dementia caregivers (Pancrazi, 2003). Pain, falls, frailty, interruption of their own medical follow-up and burn-out complaints are very common in caregivers as well (Schultz, 1999; 2000; 2004). Time dedicated to caregiving is often responsible for stopping leisure activities. Besides, the social stigmatization of people living with dementia, because of the negative representations of the disease, may lead to increased isolation of the patient and his/her caregiver (Monfort, 2006).

Psychosocial educational interventions for caregivers are available to provide information, support and counseling. Meta-analysis of several programs of this type showed their efficacy (Sorensen, 2002; Brodaty, 2003); support programs such as cognitive behavioral interventions have been showed reducing anxiety in Alzheimer's disease family caregivers (Akkerman, 2004).

The benefit of counseling for caregivers has been described by Mary Mittelman's studies since 1999 (Mittelman, 1999; 2006). In a randomized Controlled Trial (RCT) with spousal caregivers, long-term counseling – as a result - delayed the institutionalization of mild to moderately severe AD persons - when compared to usual care. The essential components of this intervention were individual assessment, information, counseling and support. Sessions of 30 to 90 min. were conducted every 2 months to twice monthly by trained personnel. The sessions focused on skill training, respite services, support groups and continuous availability of a therapist. One of these RCTs, after more than 11 years of intervention still showed a delay in nursing home placement of 557 days.

We propose to all the caregivers of people admitted in our day hospital of geriatric rehabilitation (HDJ SSR) a monthly phone support, six information meetings and training sessions. Information on the disease, its evolution and complications are given during the first three sessions while the next three sessions are dedicated to counseling and support groups. Once a month a professional calls the caregiver to give him information on the non-pharmacological interventions provided to the person with dementia and asks for needs or problems to solve. Fifty % of the caregivers accept to come to the 6 sessions offered (n=35, 2010). All of them are satisfied, and admit that a good help has been achieved. Sixty-two % admit to have learnt to better understand the symptoms, the sufferings, the expectations and the needs of their close relation and 60 % assert that these meetings restored them to hope and confidence.

The impact on caregivers is relevant - with the acquisition of new skills and know-how - allowing them to better face needs, difficulties and handicaps of their relative. They also become aware of the risks of exhaustion, psychological distress and ill-treatment. This will lead the caregiver to appeal for more human help.

The systematic attention offered by the geriatrician to caregivers is essential to prevent crises or breaks bound connected to the burn-out. The valuation of the care relation can also be gratifying to help the caregiver see its role and its position in a more positive way.

However even if caregiver support and education are essential parts in the program, interventions should be multicomponent in order to be more effective on caregiver burden and depression as shown also by the REACH multisite initiative (Gitlin, 2003).

Art Therapy

Non-pharmacological therapies can improve the quality of life of people with Alzheimer's disease and their carers. Creative activities - by offering the power of choice and decisions - are aimed to reduce depression and social isolation.

Moreover they can also improve the residual abilities of people with dementia.

As a case report showed art therapy can be beneficial for reducing stress-related behaviors in dementia (Mimica, 2011). Another paper reports the effects of a structured art program ("Memories in the Making") on the well-being, of people with dementia in the early and middle stages of the disease, compared with usual activities provided in day care centers. The results showed that during participation in the art therapy program individuals had significantly more interest, sustained attention, pleasure, self-esteem and normalcy (Kinney JM, Rentz CA, 2005)

Some other case studies report new artistic skills in people with dementia, especially people with Fronto-Temporal Dementia. Some of them never had abilities in this field before. The University of California San Francisco shows artistic productions of FTD people with dementia on its website (Liu, 2009)

On the other hand, several examples of accomplished artists who were developing dementia provided a way to explore the change in their skills. The productions of Carolus Horn, William Utermohlen, and Willem de Kooning have been studied in detail. (Crutch, 2001, Espinel, 1996)

We have 10 individual or collective art therapy sessions a week in our DCH. Twenty sessions are usually sufficient per person. Small exhibitions with people with dementia and their caregivers are organized in our unit at the end of each program. It's amazing to see how pleased and enthusiastic caregivers are by their relatives' productions and how they are discovering new perspectives. Showing their artistic productions is one of the best ways for people living with dementia to show their preserved skills or new ones and to be upgraded by their relatives. These actions improve their quality of life.

Music Therapy

The impact of music therapy on dementia is well-known (Clark,1998). Music alters the different components of the disease through sensory, cognitive, emotional, behavioral and social impacts. We have currently, 6 music therapy groups and 5 individual music therapy sessions each week in our unit. Both individual and collective sessions are improving communication skills and some behavioral symptoms like anxiety or agitation and are sometimes delaying the cognitive decline by bringing also pleasure, relaxation and cognitive stimulation as shown in the literature (Gerdner, 2000; Irish, 2006; Koger, 1999).

In the Guetin study (2009) a weekly receptive music therapy session was delivered to people with dementia over a 10-week period according to the U method standardized protocol. This technique was based on the recommendations made by Gardner and Good relating to the importance given to an individualized choice of music. Instrumental tracks were selected from various music styles (classic, jazz, world music...)

Receptive music therapy sessions specifically tailored to the needs of each person have shown to significantly reduce anxiety, depression and aggressiveness in people suffering from Alzheimer's disease. This technique has also demonstrated its impact on helping AD people recall their previous life experience. After the sessions, all people expressed a sensation of well-being and pleasure (Guetin et al, 2009). *W*e have now a one year experience with this program: 12 people with dementia have been using the method in our unit; ten of them reported a significant decrease of their anxiety at the end of the sessions. In our practice the music therapy sessions are always followed by a meeting with a nurse or a psychologist, to collect the people with dementia's feelings.

A Particular Case: Early Onset AD

The case of people with early onset AD is much more complex and need a specific think tank. These people can be taken care in the geriatric networks in France. Then they benefit from a personal and global care inherited from a long time experience in geriatrics. Unfortunately some people with early onset AD are suffering from the contact with older persons. We have also to admit that these people sometimes consulted 3 specialists before getting a diagnosis (Luscombe and Brodaty, 1998). The social representations are even more negative and people are frequently referred to the psychiatrist as if they were suffering from madness. In these persons professional, financial, family and social difficulties are piling up, which – sometimes - make them sink into an unacceptable precariousness. Their caregivers are often involved at the beginning of their professional career or if they have children, they can still be student. It is often impossible for them to provide and assure the necessary help.

Moreover the solutions of respite care are often unsuitable for early onset AD people or too difficult to access. The non-pharmacological interventions must be individualized, adapted to the age of the patient and ranked according to the priorities.

We admitted 8 people with AD aged under 65 during the last 2 years. Their stay was twice as long as late onset AD people due to social, professional, and family difficulties. We had to create individualized programs for these people and a long social follow up with the caregivers to find respite solutions. Two Respite day care centers have been created now in Paris with 2 days a week reserved for younger people with dementia which is very helpful for everyone.

Conclusion

Day Care Hospitals in France are a good answer to people with dementia and caregivers' needs and asking throughout the course of the disease. They offer non-pharmacological therapies for people with dementia and caregivers in a very supporting and appropriate place of care.

In this setting the impact of non-pharmacological therapies on caregivers is of value. Caregivers' better understanding of the disease can prevent psychobehavioral disturbances and help them to manage the situation in an appropriate way. Art therapies that are tailored to people with dementia abilities and life history - and that provide choices restore people identity - give a new look at the person and the disease and can really upgrade them. The purpose is not only to maintain autonomy as long as possible but also to improve the quality of life by reducing the psychological suffering of people with dementia and their family.

In fact several studies already showed a reduction in both the cost of care and the distress of caregivers and also a delay in nursing home placement. However non-pharmacological intervention research in AD should be conducted on a larger scale in order to establish the final scientific evidence of its effectiveness.

References

Aguglia E, Onor ML, Trevisiol M, Negro C, Saina M, Maso E. Stress in the caregivers of Alzheimer's patients: an experimental investigation in Italy. *Am. J. Alzheimers Dis Other Demen.* 2004;19(4):248-52.

Akkerman RL, Ostwald SK. Reducing anxiety in Alzheimer's disease family caregivers: the effectiveness of a nine week cognitive behavioral intervention. *Am. J. Alzheimers Dis Other Demen.* 2004, 19: 117-123.

Bonté F. Maltraitances et démences : pertinences de prise en charge en hôpital de jour psychogériatrique. NPG , *Neurologie Psychiatrie Gériatrie* ;Juin 2010.

Brodaty H, Green A, Koschera A. Meta-analysis of psychosocial interventions for caregivers of people with dementia. *J. Am. Geriatr. Soc.* 2003.51/657-64.

Brodaty H, Luscombe G . Psychological morbidity in caregivers is associated with depression in patients with dementia. *Alzheimer Dis Assoc Disord,* 1998;12(2):62-70.

Clark ME, Lipe AW, Bilbrey M. Use of music to decrease aggressive behaviors in people with dementia. *J. Gerontol. Nurs.* 1998;24:10-7.

Crutch SJ, Isaacs R, Rossor MN. Some workmen can blame their tools: artistic change in an individual with Alzheimer's disease. *Lancet* 2001; 357: 2129-33.

Espinel CH.De Kooning's late colours and forms: dementia, creativity, and the healing power of art. Lancet 1996; 347:1096-8.

Gerdner LA. Effects of individualized versus classical "relaxation" music on the frequency of agitation with Alzheimer's disease and related disorders. *Int. Psycho Geriatry* 2000;12:49-65.

Gitlin LN, Belle SH, Burgio LD, Czaja SJ, Mahonney D, Gallagher-Thompson D, and al. Effect of multicomponent interventions on caregiver burden and depression: The REACH multisite initiative at 6 month follow up. *Psychol. Aging.* 2003.18/361-74.

Guetin S, F. Portet , M.C. Picot, C. Pommié ,M. Messaoudi ,L. Djabelkir, A.L. Olsen , M.M. Cano, E. Lecourt, J. Touchon .Effect of Music Therapy on Anxiety and Depression in Patients with Alzheimer's Type Dementia: Randomised, Controlled Study. *Dement Geriatr. Cogn. Disord.* 2009;28:36–46.

INSEE: statistiques population française: www.insee.frIrish M, Cunningham CJ, Walsh JB, Coakley D, Lawlor BA, Robertson IH, Coen RF, Investigating the enhancing of music on autobiographical memory in mild Alzheimer's disease. *Dement Geriatr. Cogn. Disord.* 2006;22:108-120.

Kinney JM, Rentz CA. Observed well-being among individuals with dementia: Memories in the Making, an art program, versus other structured activity. *Am. J. Alzheimers Dis Other Demen.* 2005 Jul-Aug;20(4):220-7.

Knight BG, Lutzky SM, Macofsky-Urban F. A meta-analytic review of interventions for caregiver distress: recommendations for future research. *Gerontologist,* 1993 Apr;33(2):240-8.

Koger SM, Chapin K, Brotons M. Is music therapy an effective intervention for dementia ? A meta-analytic review of literature. *J. Music Ther.* 1999;36:2-15.

Luscombe G, Brodaty H, Freeth S. Younger people with dementia: diagnostic issues, effects on carers and use of services, *International Journal of Geriatric Psychiatry* Volume 13, Issue 5, pages 323–330, May 1998.

Liu A, Werner K, Roy S, Trojanowski JQ, Morgan-Kane U, Miller BL, Rankin KP. A case study of an emerging visual artist with frontotemporal lobar degeneration and amyotrophic lateral sclerosis ;*Neurocase.* 2009;15(3):235-47.

Mimica N, Kalinić D.Art therapy may be benefitial for reducing stress--related behaviours in people with dementia--case report.*Psychiatr. Danub.* 2011;23(1):125-8.

Mittelman M, Ferris SH, Shulman E, Steinberg G, Levin B: A family intervention to delay nursing home placement of patients with Alzheimer's disease. A randomized controlled trial . *JAMA* 1996, 276: 1725-1731.

Mittelman M, Haley WE, Clay OJ, Roth DL: Improving caregiver well-being delays nursing home placement of patients with Alzheimer's disease. *Neurology* 2006, 67: 1592-1599.

Monfort J, M.Neiss, P.Rabier, M-P Hervy. Alzheimer, Famille, Institution. Annales Médico-psychologiques,164 (2006) 726-731.

Pancrazzi MP, Metais P. La dépression des aidants familiaux dans la maladie d'Alzheimer. NPG 2003 ; 15 :16-9.

Plan Alzheimer 2008-2012 : www.plan-alzheimer.gouv.fr

Schultz R, Beach S. Caregiving as a risk factor for mortality. The caregiver health effects study. *JAMA* 1999;282:2215-19.

Schultz R, Martire LM. Family caregiving of persons with dementia: prevalence, health effects, and support strategies. *Am. J. Geriatr. Psychiatry*. 2004;12:240-9.

Schultz R, O'Brien AT, Bookwala J, Fleissner K. Psychiatric and physical morbidity effects of dementia caregiving: prevalence, correlates, and causes. *Gerontologist* , 2000; 40:147-164.

Sorensen S, Pinquart M, Duberstein PO. How effective are interventions with caregivers? An updated meta-analysis. *Gerontologist* 2002;42(3): 356-72.

Volpe-Gillot L, Bonté F . Place de l'hôpital de jour dans le diagnostic et la prise en charge de la maladie d'Alzheimer. *Soins Gerontologie*, 2008; 69 :24-26.

Wu H, Wang J, Cacioppo JT, Glaser R, Kiecolt-Glaser JK, Malarkey WB. Chronic stress associated with spousal caregiving of patients with Alzheimer's dementia is associated with downregulation of B-Lymphocyte GH mRNA. *J. Gerontol. A. Biol. Sci.,* 1999;54(4):M 212-5;

Yee JL, Schultz R. Gender. Differences in psychiatric morbidity among family caregivers. A review and analysis, *Gerontologist* 1995; 35(6):771-91.

Index

A

ABA, 100
abstraction, 87
access, x, 2, 3, 12, 16, 21, 67, 94, 99, 109, 126
accessibility, 16, 51
acetylcholinesterase, 85
acetylcholinesterase inhibitor, 85
AD, ix, 3, 17, 18, 20, 22, 23, 24, 26, 60, 73, 74, 77, 78, 79, 80, 81, 83, 84, 87, 88, 90, 106, 114, 121, 124, 125, 126
adaptation, 27, 87, 100
adjustment, 43, 60
adults, ix, 16, 32, 36, 83, 84, 91
age, ix, 4, 7, 17, 20, 45, 83, 84, 85, 88, 99, 126
aggression, 16, 43, 45, 68
aggressive behavior, 66, 127
aggressiveness, 125
agnosia, 94, 114
alertness, 42
alters, 125
American Psychiatric Association, 38
amnesia, 96, 106, 109, 111, 114
amyotrophic lateral sclerosis, 128
anterograde amnesia, 96, 111
antidepressant, 85
anxiety, 64, 66, 78, 88, 122, 123, 125, 127
apathy, 16, 45
aphasia, 3, 11, 14, 20, 106, 108, 109, 111, 114
appetite, 45
appointments, 106
arousal, 118, 119
assessment, ix, x, 13, 28, 33, 58, 66, 70, 71, 80, 83, 85, 87, 96, 113, 115, 117, 122, 124
atmosphere, 48, 49, 50, 57
atrophy, 94, 98, 109, 115, 118
attitudes, 67
attribution, 69
autobiographical memory, 109, 114, 119, 127
autonomy, 96, 106, 123, 126
awareness, 58, 74, 86, 106

B

barriers, 60
base, 35, 40, 61, 78, 90, 91, 95
batteries, 84
behavioral change, 69
behavioral manifestations, 29
behavioral problems, 69
behaviors, vii, viii, 8, 12, 15, 17, 28, 63, 64, 66, 67, 68, 69, 124, 127
Belgium, 43
beneficial effect, ix, 83
benefits, 33, 77, 78, 79
beverages, 48
blame, 127
blindness, 80
blood, 115
BPSD, viii, 28, 63, 64, 65, 67, 68, 69, 70, 123
brain, 40, 85, 96, 110, 115, 118
brain damage, 110
brothers, 3
burn, 123, 124
businesses, 123

C

caregivers, vii, viii, xi, 1, 16, 19, 25, 26, 58, 59, 60, 61, 63, 64, 65, 66, 67, 68, 69, 70, 71, 77, 78, 80, 121, 122, 123, 124, 125, 126, 127, 128
caregiving, viii, 57, 59, 63, 64, 69, 70, 123, 128
case study(s), x, 93, 96, 105, 107, 109, 119, 125, 128
categorization, 87
cell phones, 35

challenges, 33, 59
Chicago, 108
children, 91, 126
cholinesterase, ix, 73, 77, 79, 80, 81, 88, 91
cholinesterase inhibitors, ix, 73, 77, 79, 81, 88, 91
City, 34
classification, 38
clients, 44
clinical diagnosis, 88
clinical psychology, 62
clinical symptoms, 95
clinical trials, 33
cognition, 29, 32, 77, 79, 84
cognitive ability(s), 13, 88, 94
cognitive activity, 37
cognitive capacities, ix, 83, 84
cognitive deficit(s), 33, 64, 74, 85
cognitive domains, 32, 33
cognitive function, viii, ix, 31, 32, 33, 35, 42, 43, 60, 73, 77, 78, 79, 81, 83, 87, 95, 106, 107
cognitive impairment, ix, 1, 20, 32, 83, 90, 91, 95
cognitive performance, 79, 88
cognitive process, viii, 2, 31, 32, 33, 37, 74
cognitive processing, viii, 31, 32, 33, 37
cognitive profile, 86, 87
cognitive rehabilitation, ix, x, 35, 39, 73, 74, 78, 80, 81, 83, 84, 85, 88, 90, 91, 92, 109, 114, 116, 118
cognitive skills, 13, 108
cognitive stimulation, vii, ix, 17, 31, 32, 35, 43, 61, 73, 74, 77, 78, 81, 125
color, 27, 34, 97, 98, 108
combined effect, 77
communication, vii, 1, 2, 13, 14, 35, 36, 37, 53, 55, 56, 61, 67, 69, 77, 79, 80, 125
communication skills, 125
community, viii, 39, 41, 42, 48, 54, 55, 61, 64, 100
compensation, ix, 93, 100, 102, 104, 105, 106, 107
competing interests, 38
complexity, 2, 87, 115
compliance, 84
complications, 122, 124
comprehension, vii, ix, x, 1, 2, 3, 7, 8, 9, 11, 12, 13, 14, 86, 87, 93, 94, 96, 97, 98, 99, 100, 104, 105, 114, 115
computer, 50, 78, 87, 90, 91, 95, 99, 110, 119
concreteness, 108
conference, 29
confrontation, 98
consciousness, 32, 39
consensus, 39, 110, 119
consent, 4, 44, 45, 116
consolidation, 119
construction, 115
consulting, 43, 48, 52, 56, 98
contrast sensitivity, 26, 29
control group, ix, 65, 74, 77, 79, 80, 83, 85, 87, 88
controlled trials, 122
conversations, 2, 13, 14
cooking, 95, 96
cooperation, 42, 43, 51
coordination, 123
coping strategies, 66
correlation(s), 3, 17, 18, 22, 23, 29, 49, 54, 56
cost, 64, 84, 126
counseling, 69, 123, 124
creativity, 127
crises, 124
CST, 35, 78, 79
CT, 85, 98
CT scan, 85, 98
cues, x, 87, 94, 98, 99, 100, 116
culture, 98

D

daily care, 123
daily living, ix, 13, 78, 83, 86, 88, 91, 93, 95, 110
danger, 16
data analysis, 48, 103
data collection, vii, 1, 4, 8
decision task, 96, 97
declarative memory, 119
deficit, 32, 68, 98, 104, 115
degenerative dementia, 114
delirium, vii, 31, 32, 35, 37, 39, 65
delusions, 66
demographic characteristics, 86
demographic data, 85
dependent variable, 7, 8, 9, 11
depression, 2, 17, 45, 60, 61, 64, 85, 88, 122, 123, 124, 125, 127
depressive symptoms, 70, 90
designers, 19
detection, 96
deviation, 5, 9, 37, 89, 102
Diagnostic and Statistical Manual of Mental Disorders, 38
diagnostic criteria, 110
dignity, 123
direct observation, vii, 15, 27, 67, 69
disability, 45, 64, 73
discomfort, 64, 65
discrimination, 2, 115
discussion groups, 42, 48, 55
disease progression, 68
diseases, 85, 122

disorder, ix, 73, 93, 94, 114
dissatisfaction, 56
dissociation, 115
distress, 60, 64, 65, 69, 124, 126, 127
distribution, 17, 19, 24
diversity, 27
dopaminergic, 32
dosage, 33
drawing, 50, 55, 68, 114
drug therapy, 78, 81
drug treatment, 74, 80
drugs, ix, 38, 39, 73, 78, 80, 81, 85, 123
dysgraphia, 98, 103
dysphoria, 45

E

education, ix, 5, 83, 85, 88, 96, 124
educational materials, 42
educational programs, 123
elders, 39, 98, 99
emergency, 85
emotion, 43, 55, 59, 68, 69
encoding, 1
encouragement, 35, 37
energy, 26
engineering, 106
England, 38, 59, 62
enlargement, 115
environment(s), vii, 15, 16, 27, 28, 29, 35, 56, 58, 65, 67, 106
environmental conditions, 87
episodic memory, 88, 91, 94, 96, 98, 106, 115
etiology, 32
Europe, 43, 123
European Union, 123
everyday life, 84, 107
evidence, ix, 3, 12, 14, 35, 40, 57, 61, 83, 84, 88, 91, 109, 126
evidence-based program, 35
evolution, 123, 124
exclusion, 85
execution, 48
executive function, 2, 27, 32, 33, 84, 94, 96, 98
executive functioning, 2, 33
executive functions, 27, 84, 94, 96, 98
exercise, 17, 23, 24, 36, 37, 80, 86
experimental condition, 9
experimental design, 111
expertise, 42
exposure, 109, 119

F

facilitators, 60
factor analysis, 28, 64
families, viii, 13, 19, 62, 63, 64, 73, 123
family members, 4, 79, 122
family support, 59
feelings, 33, 48, 57, 125
fidelity, viii, 31, 34, 35, 36, 37
financial, 122, 126
flexibility, 16, 96
flowers, 12, 17, 19
fMRI, 118
food, x, 34, 48, 49, 95, 114, 118
football, 50
Ford, 91
formula, 17
fragments, 8
France, xi, 108, 110, 121, 122, 126
fruits, 17, 36
functional approach, 14

G

gait, 21, 66
General Health Questionnaire, 48, 60
general practitioner, xi, 48, 121
Germany, 90
gerontology, 39
gestures, 36
glasses, 36
gnosis, 78
grading, 28, 39, 70, 81, 91
graph, 101, 102, 105
group activities, 17
group therapy, 58, 61
grouping, 19
guidance, 34
guidelines, 18, 40

H

hair, 98
harmony, 19
healing, 127
health, 16, 64, 65, 81, 122, 123, 128
health care, 122
health effects, 128
hearing loss, 33
heterogeneity, 80
hippocampus, 114
history, 17, 20, 67, 86, 96, 126

hobby, 7
homeostasis, 32
homes, 28, 54, 57
homework, ix, 77, 83, 86
homogeneity, 101, 103
Hong Kong, 14
human, 40, 124
human brain, 40
hygiene, 95
hypothesis, viii, 63, 64, 65

I

ideal, ix, 83, 84
identification, x, 65, 87, 109, 113, 118
identity, 114, 126
imagery, 86
images, x, 87, 110, 113, 116
imitation, 97
impairments, 1, 33, 95
implicit memory, x, 86, 113, 114, 116, 118
improvements, 28, 64, 77, 80, 84, 90, 95
inattention, 32, 37
independence, 40, 85
individuals, vii, 2, 13, 27, 31, 32, 33, 57, 73, 84, 87, 90, 124, 127
infection, 32
inflammation, 32
information retrieval, 1
informed consent, 44, 45, 116
ingredients, 95
inhibition, 96
inhibitor, 77, 78, 79, 80
institutions, 42, 43, 44
integration, 123
interference, 48, 56, 87, 97
intervention, vii, viii, ix, x, 14, 29, 31, 32, 35, 36, 37, 38, 39, 40, 60, 61, 63, 64, 65, 66, 68, 69, 70, 73, 74, 77, 80, 84, 88, 90, 91, 93, 94, 95, 96, 98, 99, 100, 101, 102, 103, 105, 106, 107, 124, 126, 127, 128
intrinsic motivation, 33
Iowa, 71
isolation, 114, 122, 123, 124
issues, viii, 63, 64, 65, 66, 67, 69, 108, 118, 127
Italy, 43, 63, 90, 91, 113, 127

L

lack of control, 69
language impairment, 95, 108, 118
lateral sclerosis, 128
laterality, 109
lead, 106, 114, 123, 124
learning, viii, 1, 40, 63, 65, 69, 79, 86, 100, 106, 108, 110, 114, 115, 116, 118, 119
learning process, 69
leisure, 123
lesions, 85
lexical decision, 97
Likert scale, 104, 105
local community, viii, 41
localization, 115
longitudinal study, 88
long-term memory, 3, 109, 114

M

majority, viii, 26, 32, 41, 44, 45, 52, 53, 55, 56, 122
man, x, 94, 96
management, 14, 29, 43, 70, 94, 106, 107, 122, 123
Marx, v
Maryland, 39
materials, 4, 13, 42
matter, 39
MCI, ix, 83, 84, 85, 86, 87, 88, 89, 90, 92
MCSP, viii, 41, 42
measurement(s), 12, 52, 56
media, 78
medical, vii, 4, 31, 38, 42, 44, 59, 65, 66, 68, 122, 123
medication, 32
Meeting Centers Support Programme, v, viii, 41, 42, 44, 57, 58, 59
memory, ix, x, xi, 2, 3, 4, 12, 13, 14, 16, 32, 33, 34, 42, 49, 50, 78, 84, 86, 87, 90, 91, 93, 94, 96, 97, 98, 99, 104, 106, 107, 108, 109, 110, 111, 113, 114, 115, 116, 118, 119, 121, 122, 127
memory function, 96
mental state, 28, 39, 70, 81
messages, 103
meta-analysis, 57, 90, 128
metaphor, 87
misunderstanding, 115
mobile phone, 106, 110
models, 74
morbidity, 127, 128
mortality, 122, 128
motivation, x, 33, 35, 37, 114, 118
motor behavior, 66
motor control, 96, 98
MRI, 116
mRNA, 128
multidimensional, 74
multimedia, 78, 81

museums, 50
music, 17, 42, 49, 55, 121, 122, 125, 127
music therapy, 121, 125, 127

N

naming, ix, x, 93, 94, 95, 96, 97, 98, 99, 100, 104, 105, 110, 114, 115, 116, 118, 119
narratives, 3
National Institutes of Health, 38
negative consequences, 123
negative relation, 68, 69
neglect, 4
neocortex, 109, 114
Netherlands, 41, 43, 44
neurodegeneration, 64
neurodegenerative disorders, 107
neuroleptic drugs, 39
neurological rehabilitation, ix, 73
neuropsychological tests, ix, 83, 84, 96, 97
neuroscience, 108, 111
neutral, 18, 95
New England, 38
nursing, 2, 3, 4, 14, 27, 28, 33, 35, 39, 40, 42, 43, 45, 47, 57, 58, 60, 61, 124, 126, 128
nursing care, 27
nursing home, 2, 3, 14, 28, 33, 35, 39, 40, 43, 45, 47, 57, 58, 60, 61, 124, 126, 128

O

oil, 28
opportunities, 16, 19, 48, 55
optimal performance, 13
organic disease, 68
organize, 35

P

pagers, 35
pain, 36, 65
parents, 45
participants, viii, 12, 33, 35, 37, 41, 44, 45, 47, 48, 49, 50, 51, 53, 55, 56, 85, 86, 88
pathology, 69, 123
pathophysiology, 32
pathways, 16, 19, 122
PCA, 61
personal control, 65
personal problems, 52, 56
personal relations, 69
personal relationship, 69
personality, 69
personality traits, 69
PET, 98, 109
PET scan, 98
pharmacological therapies, vii, xi, 80, 121, 122, 124, 126
pharmacological treatment, vii, ix, 73, 74, 77, 78, 79, 80, 84
pharmacotherapy, 122
Philadelphia, 39
photographs, 3, 4, 11, 12, 13, 86
physical environment, 28
physical exercise, 17, 23, 24
physical function, vii, 31, 32, 33
physical health, 16, 123
physical therapist, 110
pilot study, ix, 3, 29, 40, 80, 81, 83, 84, 108
pitch, 36
placebo, 28
plants, 19, 27
plasticity, 40, 60
playing, 17, 49
pleasure, 124, 125
PM, 38
population, 3, 26, 32, 37, 71, 87, 90, 91, 106, 127
positive emotions, 33
praxis, 95
preparation, 43, 98
presentation order, 5
preservation, 13, 111
principles, 35, 115
problem behavior(s), 66
problem solving, 87
procedural memory, 106
professionalism, 53, 56
professionals, 13, 42, 43, 122, 123
prognosis, 88
project, 37, 48
prosthesis, 16
psychiatric disorders, 28
psychiatric illness, 4
psychiatric morbidity, 128
psychiatrist, 126
psychoeducational intervention, 122
psychoeducational program, 123
psychological distress, 64, 124
psychological problems, 48
psychological well-being, 59, 69
psychologist, 66, 67, 68, 69, 122, 125
psychology, 13, 39, 62
psychopathology, 28, 58, 70
psychopharmacology, 61
psychosis, vii, 15, 17, 18

psychosocial factors, 58
psychosocial interventions, 60, 61, 69, 127
psychosomatic, 44, 45
psychotic symptoms, 28

Q

qualitative differences, 12
quality of life, 2, 13, 19, 43, 60, 64, 73, 84, 114, 118, 122, 123, 124, 125, 126
quality standards, 29
questionnaire, 19, 25, 45, 47, 48, 49, 50, 51, 52, 53, 56, 66, 67, 68, 115

R

rating scale, 81
reaction time, 86
reactions, 68
reading, vii, 1, 2, 3, 4, 5, 7, 8, 9, 10, 11, 12, 13, 14, 17, 42, 49, 97
reading accuracy, vii, 1, 2, 3, 8
reading comprehension, vii, 1, 2, 3, 8, 9, 11, 13, 14
reading skills, 2
real time, 98
reality, 43, 55, 77, 87
reality orientation, 43, 77, 87
reasoning, 90
recall, 85, 86, 88, 89, 90, 98, 100, 102, 115, 125
recognition, 96, 97, 114
recognition phase, 96
recommendations, 125, 127
recovery, 32
recreation, 35, 39, 40, 96, 98
recreational, vii, 31, 32, 33, 39, 40
rehabilitation, vii, ix, x, xi, 29, 35, 36, 39, 66, 71, 73, 74, 78, 80, 81, 83, 84, 85, 86, 87, 88, 90, 91, 92, 93, 94, 96, 99, 108, 109, 111, 113, 114, 116, 117, 118, 121, 122, 123, 124
rehabilitation program, ix, 83, 84, 85, 86, 88, 91, 92, 117, 118
reinforcement, 78
relatives, x, 19, 25, 27, 78, 85, 113, 114, 115, 117, 118, 125
relaxation, 125, 127
relevance, 95, 107, 122
reliability, 17, 18, 33, 91
remediation, 39
repetitions, 11
replication, 13
reproduction, 114
requirements, 99
researchers, 3, 48, 77
Residential, 14
resistance, 27
resolution, 37, 122, 123
resources, 86, 87, 118
response, 2, 6, 36, 39, 122
rings, 4
risk(s), vii, 17, 29, 31, 32, 56, 64, 84, 122, 124, 128
risk management, 29
Rouleau, 105, 110
routes, 87
routines, 14, 86
rules, 70, 91

S

safety, 16, 17, 19, 67
science, 99
sclerosis, 128
scope, 86
security, 16, 67
selective attention, 87
self-confidence, 68, 69
self-efficacy, 64, 65
self-esteem, 43, 124
self-reports, 100, 104
semantic information, x, 94, 96, 103, 105, 114
semantic memory, ix, 3, 93, 94, 96, 98, 99, 106, 107, 108, 109, 110, 115, 119
semantic processing, 98
senile dementia, 60
sensation, 125
sensitivity, 26, 29
sensory impairments, 33
sentence comprehension, 2
services, 51, 62, 93, 124, 127
sex, 45
shape, 26, 34
showing, 79, 90
significance level, 49
signs, 87, 97
social activities, vii, 15, 19, 23
social behaviour, 43
social care, 81
social desirability, 106
social interactions, 2
social network, 44
social stigmatization, 123
social support, viii, 41, 42
social withdrawal, 2
socialization, 2
society, 74
software, 85, 106
specialists, xi, 121, 122, 126

species, 20
speech, 8, 42, 65, 94, 97, 114, 115, 122
spelling, 3, 97
spelling to dictation, 97
spirituality, 65
Spring, 44
stability, 13
stabilization, 88, 102
staff members, 16, 18, 19, 25, 26, 48
standard deviation, 5, 9, 89, 102
stars, 34
state(s), 25, 28, 31, 39, 70, 81, 91
statistics, 48, 67
stimulation, vii, ix, 16, 17, 19, 27, 31, 32, 35, 39, 43, 57, 61, 66, 73, 74, 77, 78, 80, 81, 86, 116, 125
stimulus, vii, 1, 3, 7, 11, 12
storage, 109
stress, viii, 16, 57, 59, 63, 64, 65, 66, 67, 68, 70, 122, 124, 128
stroke, 29, 71
stupor, 32
subgroups, 61, 74
support services, 51
surgical conditions, vii, 31
surplus, 57
survivors, 32
symptoms, viii, 17, 28, 29, 33, 39, 44, 45, 49, 50, 54, 55, 60, 61, 63, 64, 70, 77, 78, 84, 88, 95, 110, 111, 122, 123, 124, 125
syndrome, 32, 51, 119

T

target, ix, 18, 25, 32, 64, 69, 83, 84, 87, 95, 103, 107, 123
target identification, 87
task difficulty, 35, 36
techniques, x, 35, 86, 113, 114, 115, 116, 117, 118
technology(s), ix, x, 93, 94, 95, 96, 106, 107, 118, 119
telephone, 52, 54, 56, 95
temperature, 17, 18, 26
temporal lobe, 94, 98, 109
tension, 16
testing, 27, 37, 86
therapeutic protocol, vii, 15
therapeutics, 122
therapist, 42, 66, 96, 98, 100, 102, 122, 124
therapy, xi, 17, 28, 33, 35, 40, 43, 49, 58, 60, 61, 65, 78, 79, 81, 95, 106, 107, 108, 111, 118, 121, 124, 125, 127, 128
Toyota, 110
tracks, 125
training, viii, x, 14, 33, 39, 40, 42, 57, 63, 70, 74, 79, 80, 81, 84, 86, 87, 88, 90, 96, 100, 102, 103, 106, 110, 111, 113, 114, 116, 117, 118, 119, 123, 124
training programs, 86
traits, 69
transcripts, 8
transient ischemic attack, 4
transmission, 32
transport, 35
transportation, 53, 56
treatment, vii, viii, ix, 28, 29, 31, 32, 34, 35, 36, 37, 43, 45, 47, 58, 61, 73, 74, 77, 79, 80, 83, 84, 85, 95, 108, 110, 119, 122, 124
trial, 29, 39, 57, 61, 70, 81, 84, 128

U

UK, 31, 58, 70, 81, 108, 109, 110

V

validation, 70
valuation, 65, 124, 123
variables, 7, 8, 9, 11, 17, 48, 88, 106
variations, 45, 58
vascular dementia, 4
vegetables, x, 19, 113, 116, 117, 118
ventricle, 115
verbal fluency, ix, 83, 85, 89
vision, 2, 26, 33, 35, 69
visual images, 86
visual stimuli, 2, 3
vocabulary, x, 4, 106, 109, 113, 114, 117, 119
vocational training, 123

W

Wales, 31
walking, 17, 42, 50, 55
wants and needs, 2
Washington, 14, 38
websites, 103
welfare, 16, 42, 43, 57
well-being, 59, 69, 124, 125, 127, 128
wellness, 19
windows, 26, 106
withdrawal, 2
wood, 34, 42
word meanings, 99
workers, 79
working memory, 97
worldwide, 73
writing to dictation, 97